NEW
KETO
COOKING

NEW KETO COOKING

Fresh Ideas
for Delicious
Low-Carb Meals
at Home

MICHAEL SILVERSTEIN

Featured on
MasterChef Season 10

PAGE STREET
PUBLISHING CO.

PAGE STREET
PUBLISHING CO.

First published in 2020 by
Page Street Publishing Co.
27 Congress Street, Suite 105
Salem, MA 01970
www.pagestreetpublishing.com

Distributed by Macmillan, sales in Canada by The Canadian Manda Group.

24   23   22   21   20   1   2   3   4   5

ISBN-13: 978-1-64567-158-9
ISBN-10: 1-64567-158-5

Library of Congress Control Number: 2019957322

Cover and book design by Molly Gillespie for Page Street Publishing Co.
"Chef Michael" Logo Design by Tess Kamban
Photography by Michael Silverstein
Author portraits by B. Moore

Printed and bound in China

Page Street Publishing protects our planet by donating to nonprofits like The Trustees, which focuses on local land conservation.

THIS BOOK IS FOR JACOB

The man who inspires me to do better and be better;
the person who pushes me to follow my dreams.
Without him, none of this would be possible.

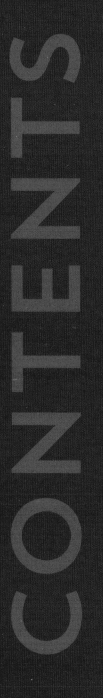

CONTENTS

Introduction   8

Cook like a Pro   10

BRUNCH WITH FRIENDS   12

Asparagus & Goat Cheese Frittata   14

Stacked Breakfast Tostadas   17

Parmesan Prosciutto Tartlets   18

Spicy Sausage & Feta Shakshuka   21

Butternut Squash & Chorizo Hash   22

LUNCH YOU'LL LOVE   24

Shrimp Fajitas with Chipotle Crema   26

Bangkok Chicken Satay with Peanut Sauce   29

Spiced Lamb Meatballs   30

Hearty Grilled Steak & Kale Salad   33

Vietnamese "Banh Mi" Lettuce Wraps   34

Boursin-Stuffed Chicken   37

INSPIRED WEEKNIGHT MEALS   38

Rosemary Dijon Chicken & Haricots Verts   40

Mediterranean Roasted Salmon & Brussels Sprouts   43

Seared Ribeye with Blue Cheese & Chive Compound Butter   44

Lemon Caper Shrimp & Avocado   47

Miso-Glazed Pork Ribs   48

Juicy Argentinean Skirt Steak & Chimichurri   51

The Chicken-Bacon-Mushroom Skillet   52

Slow Cooker Carnitas with Ancho Chile   55

Salmon Croquettes with Turmeric-Ginger Aioli   56

Creamy Sun-Dried Tomato Chicken   59

Grilled Chicken Shawarma with Dill Yogurt Sauce   60

Pork Chops with Creamy Mushroom Sauce   63

Korean BBQ Pork Belly   64

Instant Pot Paneer Korma   67

DINNERS TO IMPRESS   68

Mike's Signature Crab Cakes   70

Secret-Recipe Whole Roasted Chicken   73

Crispy-Skin Salmon with Brown Butter & Pancetta   74

Filet Mignon with Warm Spinach & Balsamic Reduction   77

Roasted Lamb Rack with Creamy Feta Sauce   78

Cod with Charred Lemon & Braised Leeks   81

Black Pepper Braised Short Ribs   82

Seared Scallops with Pea Puree & Prosciutto Crisps   85

Moroccan Chicken Tagine 86

Korean Beef Bulgogi Ssam 89

Seared Snapper with
Wine-Braised Red Cabbage 90

Za'atar-Crusted Chicken &
Roasted Carrots 93

Spice-Rubbed Pork Tenderloin
with Orange Gastrique 94

VEGGIES & SIDES 96

Grilled Asparagus with
Feta & Pistachio 98

The Perfect Mashed
"Faux-tatoes" 101

Cheesy Brussels Sprout Gratin 102

Herb-Roasted Kabocha Squash 105

Lemony Charred Broccolini 106

The Ultimate Creamy "Risotto" 109

Button Mushroom Flambé 110

Jicama & Orange Slaw 113

SWEET TREATS 114

Berry Cheesecake Trifle 116

Spiced Carrot Cake with
Cardamom Cream Cheese
Frosting 119

Caramel Flan with Candy Tuile 120

Strawberry Balsamic Ice Cream 123

Key Lime Cheesecake 124

Fluffy "Churro" Donuts 127

Chocolate Peanut Butter Pie 128

Buttery Ghee Pound Cake 131

Tres Leches Cupcakes with
Cinnamon Whipped Frosting 132

Tiramisu Mousse 135

EASY SAUCES &
MARINADES 136

Spicy Red Chimichurri 138

Garlic Aioli
(The Best Mayo from Scratch) 141

Avocado Salsa Verde 142

Secret-Ingredient Cheese
Sauce 145

Meyer Lemon Vinaigrette 146

Easy Tahini Yogurt Sauce 149

Japanese Sesame Ginger
Dressing 150

Zesty Dill Rémoulade 153

Cinnamon Caramel Sauce 154

References 156

Acknowledgments 158

About the Author 161

Index 162

INTRODUCTION

As a chef and true lover of food, it is so important to me that I bring you a fresh approach to Keto, one that reimagines healthy cuisine. Instead of falling back on the typical "diet" substitutions, the unique recipes in this book have been carefully developed to feature big, bold flavors. My goal is to show you how easy it is to create restaurant-quality food at home, whether for your family, a date night or your next dinner party. And to keep things simple and approachable, each recipe has been crafted to use only common supermarket ingredients. I want to make Keto food exciting, and I hope to inspire you to try something new in the kitchen.

I've loved cooking my entire life, and this book is a culmination of everything I have learned. From my first job in an Italian restaurant at thirteen years old, the kitchen has been euphoric to me. I started by clearing tables, filling water glasses and building rapport with the kitchen staff. Soon, the chefs were sneaking me lessons in making the sauces, searing the meat and composing the dishes. And although I would end up working at many restaurants over the next decade, it was then that I knew I wanted to cook.

Traveling has also become a huge source of culinary inspiration for me, and you'll see that throughout the book. I have such distinct memories wandering the endless aisles of street-food carts in Thailand and the spice markets of India. I'll never forget the elder woman in a small seaside village in South Korea pulling a live fish out of the water and carving it into exquisite sashimi on a plastic folding table. In Seoul, I remember sitting cross-legged on the floor as a woman sliced a live octopus and taught me how to eat it so I didn't choke on its still-moving tentacles. These moments sparked something inside me that will never be extinguished: a true love for exploring the world of food. I learned how important it is to take risks in the kitchen, and I hope you'll do the same.

While food has been a constant source of happiness in my life, it did come at a cost. I steadily gained weight through my twenties, and by age thirty, worried about my health, I decided to make a change. I knew that I could never suppress my love for food, and more important, I didn't want to. I researched diets that weren't based on counting calories or "points," knowing I had to find a way to continue enjoying food, but with structure. I discovered the Ketogenic diet, and through research, started realizing the whole-health benefits of the lifestyle. Within days of eliminating sugar, I felt better. My energy levels skyrocketed and the stomachaches disappeared. That year, I lost just over 80 pounds (36 kg) by cooking within the low-carb, high-fat framework. I developed a passion for writing beautiful Keto recipes and launched my career as a recipe developer.

In the fall of 2018, I was asked to go to New York City to cook for one of Gordon Ramsay's chefs. This was the start of a completely unexpected journey to television. The first dish I presented to the judge was a sous-vide duck breast with roasted golden beets, celery root puree (try it on page 101!) and basil aioli. When Gordon's chef whispered, "You knocked it out of the park," I was on my way to Hollywood. *MasterChef* became an unforgettable adventure and profoundly challenged me to learn and grow as a chef.

Writing a cookbook has been a dream come true, and I feel unimaginably grateful to be here, sharing these recipes with you and inviting you into my kitchen. I hope that this book serves as a means of discovering your own culinary passion, just as much a tool to use on your journey to health. Food is my world, and I thank you for letting me share that with you. Now, roll up your sleeves and let's get cooking!

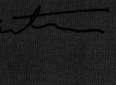

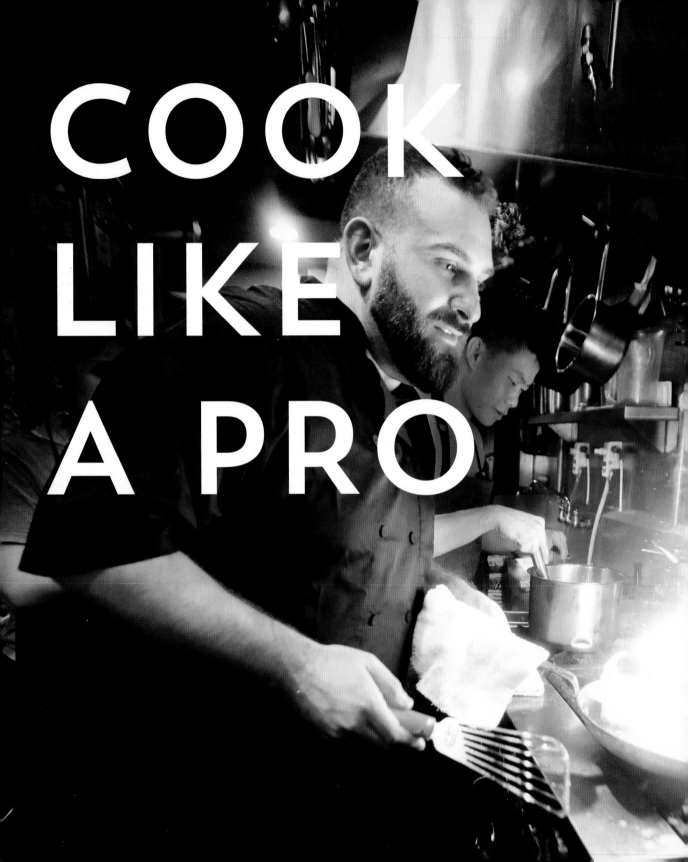

COOK
LIKE
A PRO

Here are a few of my tricks of the trade to help you cook at home with ease and confidence. I've also snuck in a few detailed "Pro Tips" in the recipes throughout the book. I want you to master your kitchen and love the food you're making.

Salt is key: Generously salting (or "seasoning") your food is absolutely essential. Understanding how and when to use various types of salt is the easiest way to cook like a pro. To ensure every recipe is perfectly salted, this book uses only Morton's kosher salt. Learn why in the "Salt Guide" (page 156).

Fat is your friend: Learning the various oils and their smoke points (what temperature they burn at) is critical. Check out the "Cooking Fats & Oils" guide (page 157) for more info.

Implement mise en place: French for "put in place," do all of your prep work for a dish, such as chopping, peeling and measuring, before you start cooking. This way, you can focus on cook times and techniques while making the recipe.

Temp your meats: Use a meat thermometer for perfectly cooked meat every single time. See the "Meat Temperature Guide" (page 157) for details.

Practice plating: We eat with our eyes first, so try plating your dishes. You can have elevated food at home, and plating certainly helps you do that. It's also a great way to support portion control.

Travel, near and far: Check out your local farmers' markets, take a road trip or even travel abroad. Exploration can be an incredible source of culinary inspiration.

Have fun in the kitchen: Don't be afraid to experiment and put your own spin on these recipes. And be sure to make cooking the best part of your day. Pour a glass of wine, play some music and make it something you look forward to.

BRUNCH
with FRIENDS

WE ALL KNOW HOW BUSY LIFE CAN GET, WHICH is why I love a good Sunday brunch. It's a great time to just slow down, invite a few friends over and make some mimosas. These elevated breakfast dishes are designed to please a crowd and are easy enough to make ahead, so you can sit back and enjoy your Sunday, too!

Asparagus & Goat Cheese Frittata (page 14)

Stacked Breakfast Tostadas (page 17)

Parmesan Prosciutto Tartlets (page 18)

Spicy Sausage & Feta Shakshuka (page 21)

Butternut Squash & Chorizo Hash (page 22)

10 large eggs

2 large egg yolks

½ cup (120 ml) heavy whipping cream

1 tsp kosher salt

½ tsp freshly ground black pepper

2 tsp (1 g) herbes de Provence

¼ cup (25 g) grated Parmesan cheese

¼ cup (57 g or ½ stick) unsalted butter, melted

8 oz (225 g) asparagus, cut into ½" (1.3-cm) slices

4 oz (115 g) goat or feta cheese, crumbled

Nonstick cooking spray

MACROS *per* SERVING

Calories: 365 • Fat: 32.1 g

Carbs: 3.2 g • Net Carbs: 2 g

Protein: 16.9 g

ASPARAGUS & GOAT CHEESE FRITTATA

This French-inspired frittata is absolutely delightful. It's ideal for entertaining, since you can make it ahead and just warm it up when guests arrive. The herbs and creamy goat cheese bring complexity and sophistication to the dish (and if you don't like goat cheese, feta works well here, too). Pair this with a simple arugula salad, some shaved Parmesan and a Bloody Mary for the perfect brunch.

Preheat your oven to 325°F (170°C). In a large bowl, combine the eggs, yolks and cream. Whisk the mixture really well, until it's velvety smooth. Then, stir in the salt, pepper, herbes de Provence, Parmesan and melted butter. Add the sliced asparagus and crumbled cheese, and stir gently.

Place a 10-inch (25-cm) ovenproof, nonstick pan over high heat. Lightly spray with cooking spray. Once hot, pour in the egg mixture. Do not stir. Simply leave it on the heat for exactly 2 minutes. Then, carefully place the entire pan in the oven. Cook the frittata for 25 minutes, or until the center is just set. (You can tell by lightly shaking the pan. If the center is jiggly, it's not ready.) Remove it from the oven and serve.

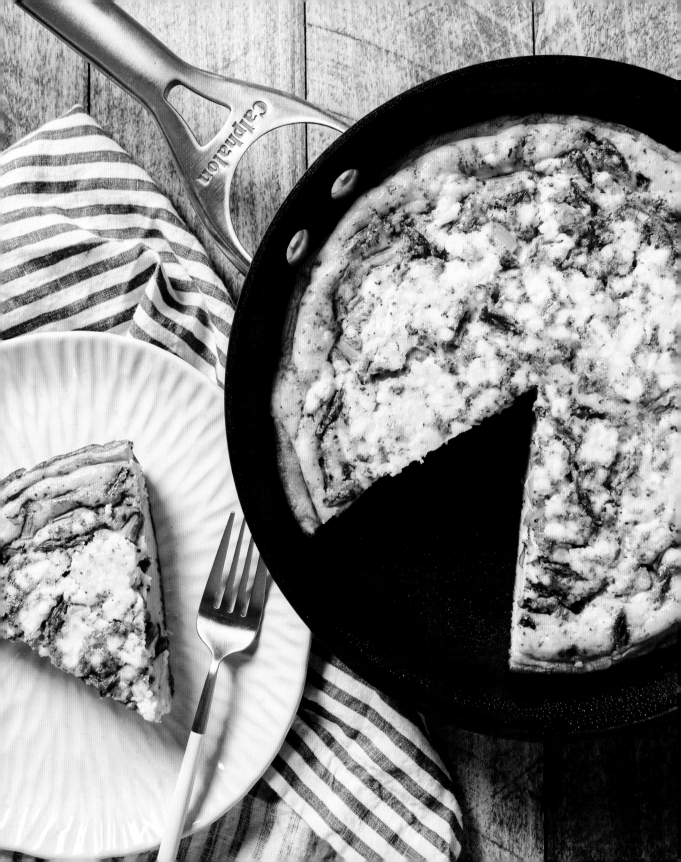

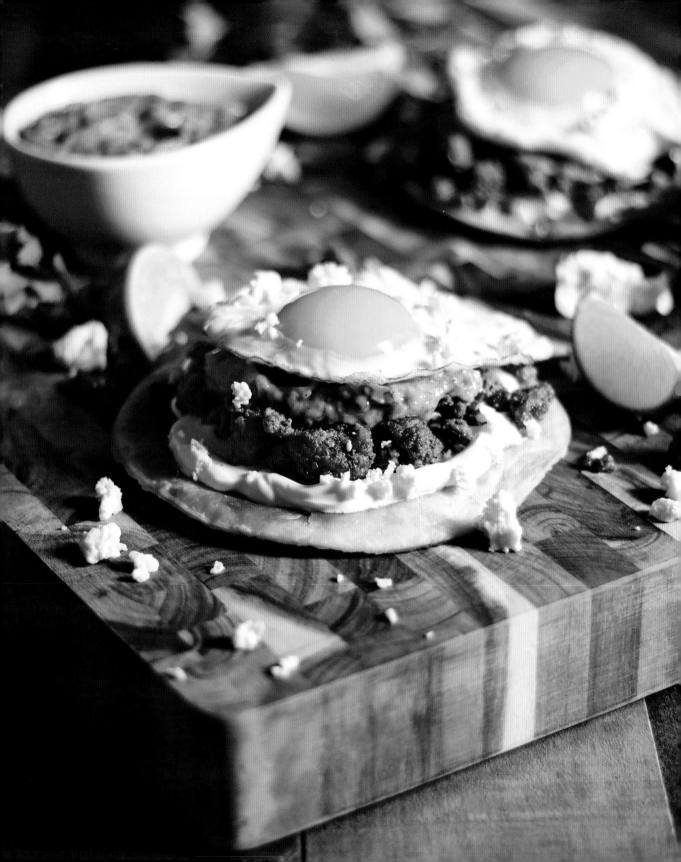

4 low-carb tortillas

2 tbsp (30 ml) avocado oil

1 lb (455 g) ground beef

1 tsp garlic powder

1 tsp kosher salt

¼ tsp freshly ground black pepper

¼ tsp ground cumin

2 tbsp (28 g) unsalted butter

4 large eggs

¼ cup (60 g) sour cream

1 batch Avocado Salsa Verde (page 142) or your favorite salsa

1 oz (28 g) queso fresco

Lime wedges, for garnish (optional)

MACROS *per* SERVING

Calories: 596 ● Fat: 42.5 g

Carbs: 11.7 g ● Net Carbs: 6.1 g

Protein: 39.8 g

STACKED BREAKFAST TOSTADAS

This yummy "stacked" breakfast is inspired by a hole-in-the-wall breakfast restaurant in Mexico that I fell in love with. Every day, the owner would cook up the most delicious food, and I was always impressed by the simplicity of her cooking. Crispy tortillas, seasoned beef and lots of toppings make for the tastiest way to start the day.

Cut the tortillas into 5-inch (13.5-cm) rounds by using a bowl to trace around with a knife. Then, in a skillet placed over medium-high heat, heat the avocado oil and fry the tortillas, one at a time, for about 1 minute on each side, or until they're golden brown and crispy.

In a large, nonstick pan over high heat, sauté the ground beef along with the garlic powder, salt, pepper and cumin for about 3 minutes. Once cooked, set the beef aside in a bowl.

In a large, nonstick skillet over medium-high heat, heat the butter. Once it has melted, carefully crack the eggs into the hot pan (avoid breaking the yolks). Fry the eggs for about 3 minutes, or until the whites are cooked but the yolks are still soft, then turn off the heat.

Assemble the tostadas by placing a crispy tortilla on each of four plates. Then, spread them with the sour cream. Add a layer of ground beef, then salsa, and finally top with a fried egg. Top with crumbled queso fresco and garnish with lime wedges (if using). I like to serve it family style on a large cutting board.

Nonstick cooking spray

6 slices prosciutto (3 oz [85 g])

6 large eggs

3 tbsp (15 g) shredded Parmesan cheese

⅛ tsp freshly ground black pepper

6 fresh basil leaves

MACROS *per* SERVING

Calories: 237 • Fat: 12.4 g

Carbs: 1 g • Net Carbs: 1 g

Protein: 21.1 g

PARMESAN PROSCIUTTO TARTLETS

This brunch meal couldn't be easier, and it's designed for a crowd. While these little egg bites may seem simple, the Italian flavors bring a sophisticated edge to breakfast with the crispy prosciutto and fresh basil.

Preheat your oven to 375°F (190°C) and spray six wells of a muffin pan with cooking spray. Line the muffin pan with slices of prosciutto. It's okay if the prosciutto sticks out of each muffin tin around the edges as it will crisp up and look pretty after it bakes. Crack an egg in each of the six spots, ensuring you don't break the yolks. Then sprinkle about ½ tablespoon (3 g) of Parmesan over each tartlet. Next, top with the pepper. Bake for 10 minutes (for a runny yolk) or 12 minutes (for a more set yolk).

While the tartlets bake, chiffonade the basil (cut into fine "ribbons"). Once they are done, remove the tartlets from the oven and let them rest for 5 minutes to cool down. Carefully remove the tartlets from the muffin pan and top with the basil chiffonade.

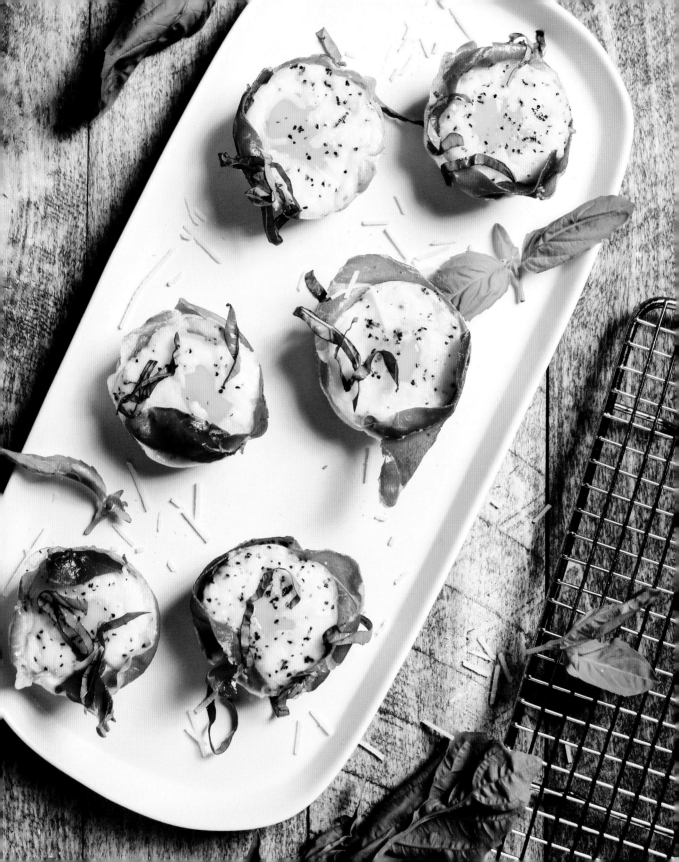

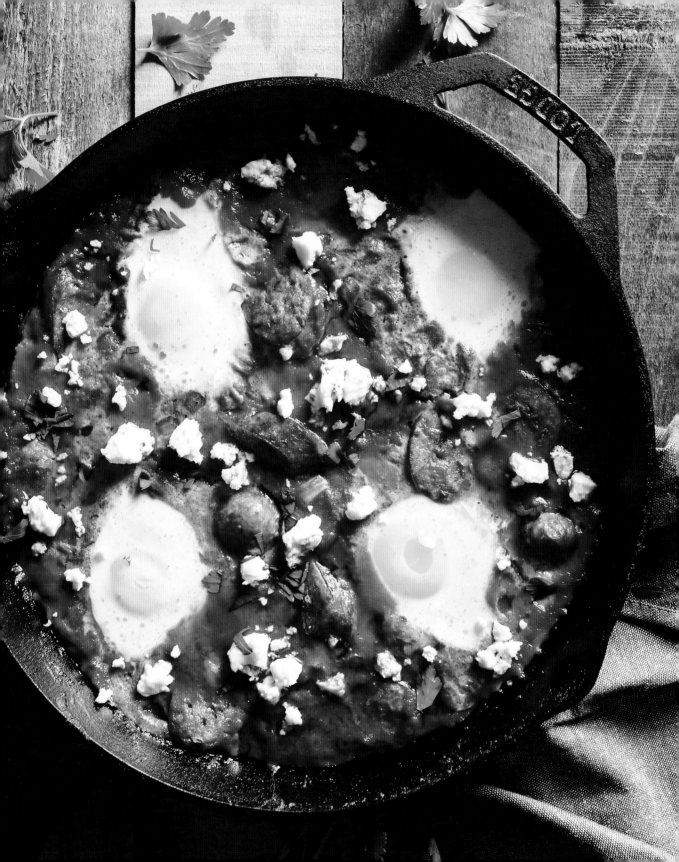

3 links spicy Italian sausage

2 tbsp (30 ml) olive oil

1 yellow onion, chopped

1 red bell pepper, seeded and chopped

3 tbsp (21 g) paprika

½ tsp ground cumin

⅛ tsp ground cinnamon

¼ tsp freshly ground black pepper

1 tbsp (6 g) finely chopped garlic

1 tbsp (16 g) tomato paste

24 oz (680 g) no-sugar-added marinara sauce

4 large eggs

2 oz (55 g) feta, crumbled

Fresh parsley, roughly chopped, for garnish (optional)

MACROS *per* SERVING

Calories: 381 • Fat: 38.4 g

Carbs: 14.6 g • Net Carbs: 12.2 g

Protein: 25.1 g

SPICY SAUSAGE & FETA SHAKSHUKA

A breakfast staple in Israel and the Middle East, this shakshuka is full of warm spices that will truly light up your taste buds. The rich tomato sauce is balanced by the gooey eggs and creamy feta. If you are looking to spice up your breakfast table, this is the recipe for you.

Preheat your oven to 350°F (180°C). In a large, cast-iron skillet over medium-high heat, sauté the sausage links for about 4 minutes. Be sure to rotate them to get some color on all sides. The sausage does not need to be cooked through, this is just to develop color and flavor. Remove the sausages from the pan and slice them into ¼-inch (6-mm) slices.

Place the same cast-iron pan over high heat. Add the olive oil and sauté the onion and bell pepper for about 4 minutes, or until they are cooked through. It's okay if the edges get a bit charred, as the smoky flavor will only enhance the dish. Once cooked, lower the heat to low and add the paprika, cumin, cinnamon, black pepper, garlic and tomato paste. Stir well for about 1 full minute to toast the spices. Then, add the marinara. Scrape the bottom of the pan to remove the fond (fond is the browned bits stuck to the bottom of the pan, and it is packed with flavor!), and stir well to combine everything.

Add the partially cooked sausage back to the pan and gently stir. Then, crack the eggs directly on top of the mixture (try to keep the yolks from breaking). Transfer the pan to the oven and bake for 10 to 12 minutes (depending on how runny you like the yolk).

Remove from the oven, and while still hot, sprinkle the top with crumbled feta and parsley, to garnish (if using).

1 lb (455 g) butternut squash, peeled, seeded and cubed (I buy it prechopped)

1 large yellow onion, chopped

1 green bell pepper, seeded and chopped

1 tbsp (15 ml) olive oil

1½ tsp (9 g) kosher salt, plus more for eggs

¼ tsp freshly ground black pepper

8 oz (225 g) uncooked tube chorizo

4 large eggs

Fresh cilantro, for garnish (optional)

Crumbled queso fresco, for garnish (optional)

MACROS *per* SERVING

Calories: 347 • Fat: 24.2 g

Carbs: 20.3 g • Net Carbs: 15.2 g

Protein: 15.3 g

BUTTERNUT SQUASH & CHORIZO HASH

This unexpected combination brings some spice to breakfast by using traditional Latin-style chorizo. Find the chorizo in the fridge case near the bacon at your grocery store. The recipe only has a few ingredients, each one full of exciting flavors. Once you cut the runny egg over it, magic happens.

Preheat your oven to 400°F (200°C). Heat a large, cast-iron skillet over high heat. Add the veggies, olive oil, salt and black pepper, and sauté for about 10 minutes, or until fork-tender.

Meanwhile, in a nonstick pan over medium-high heat, sauté the chorizo for about 5 minutes. Once cooked, mix the chorizo into the vegetable hash. (If the chorizo pan has a lot of grease in it, use a slotted spoon to remove the chorizo, leaving the grease behind.) Then, pour the hash onto a rimmed baking sheet. Avoiding breaking the yolks, crack the eggs over the top of the hash. Transfer the pan to the oven and bake for about 15 minutes, or until the eggs have cooked. Garnish with cilantro and a sprinkle of crumbled queso fresco (if using).

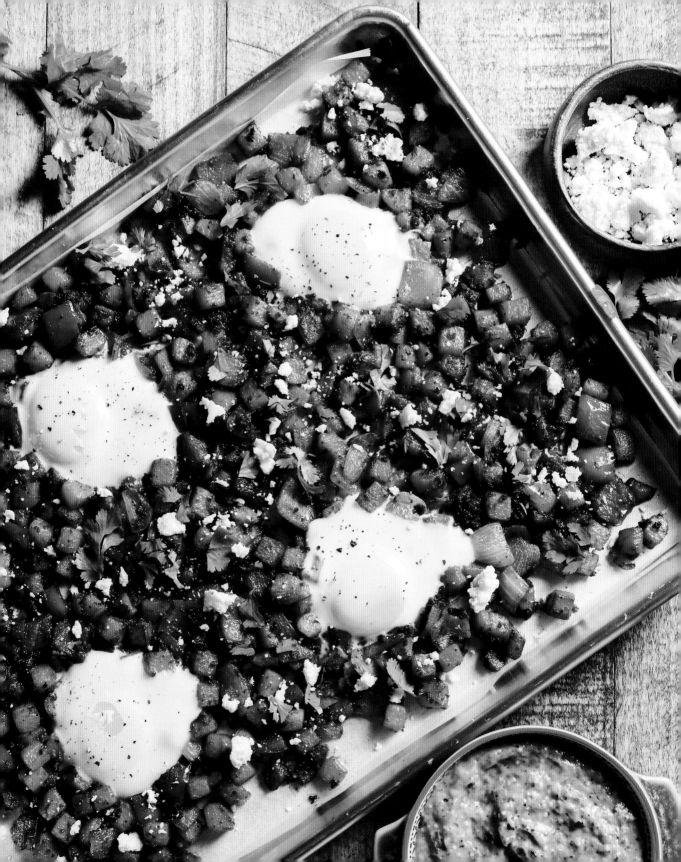

LUNCH
you'll LOVE

PREPARING LUNCHES FOR THE WEEK IS SUCH A NICE way to ensure you're eating well, even at work (it saves money, too!). And these meals keep lunch way more interesting. Leave the turkey sandwich at home and try these fun and healthy dishes instead.

Shrimp Fajitas with Chipotle Crema (page 26)

Bangkok Chicken Satay with Peanut Sauce (page 29)

Spiced Lamb Meatballs (page 30)

Hearty Grilled Steak & Kale Salad (page 33)

Vietnamese "Banh Mi" Lettuce Wraps (page 34)

Boursin-Stuffed Chicken (page 37)

½ cup (115 g) sour cream

1 (3.5-oz [100-g]) can chipotle peppers in adobo, peppers and sauce separated

1 red bell pepper, seeded and stemmed

1 yellow bell pepper, seeded and stemmed

1 yellow or white onion

1 lb (455 g) shrimp, thawed, peeled and deveined

1 tbsp (15 ml) avocado oil

1 tsp ground cumin

1 tsp garlic powder

1 tsp kosher salt

Juice of 1 lime

Chopped fresh cilantro, for garnish (optional)

MACROS *per* SERVING

Calories: 190 • Fat: 8.7 g

Carbs: 8.5 g • Net Carbs: 7.4 g

Protein: 16.8 g

SHRIMP FAJITAS WITH CHIPOTLE CREMA

I love going to a Mexican restaurant and watching as the sizzling fajita plate comes over to the table. This recipe brings all the flavors of classic fajitas, but quickly and easily at home. This makes for the perfect low-carb lunch, but it's a great easy dinner as well. And the addition of a simple two-ingredient chipotle crema adds heat and creaminess to the dish.

First, make the sauce by mixing the sour cream with only the sauce from the can of chipotle peppers in adobo (you need 1 to 2 teaspoons [5 to 10 ml] of adobo sauce, depending on how spicy you want it). Save the chipotle peppers in the can for another recipe (like the Spicy Red Chimichurri, page 138).

Next, slice the bell peppers and onion into ¼-inch (6-mm)-wide strips. Make sure your shrimp is thawed and pat them dry with a paper towel.

Heat a large, cast-iron skillet over high heat. You want it to be smoking hot. Add the avocado oil, bell peppers and onion to the pan. Cook over high heat for about 5 minutes. Do not overstir the veggies, as you want them to char and get a nice color. Then, add the cumin, garlic powder, salt and shrimp to the pan. Stir to combine and sauté for another 3 minutes, or just until the shrimp curls up and turns opaque. Finish with the fresh lime juice.

Plate the fajitas with a drizzle of the chipotle sauce on top and some chopped cilantro (if using).

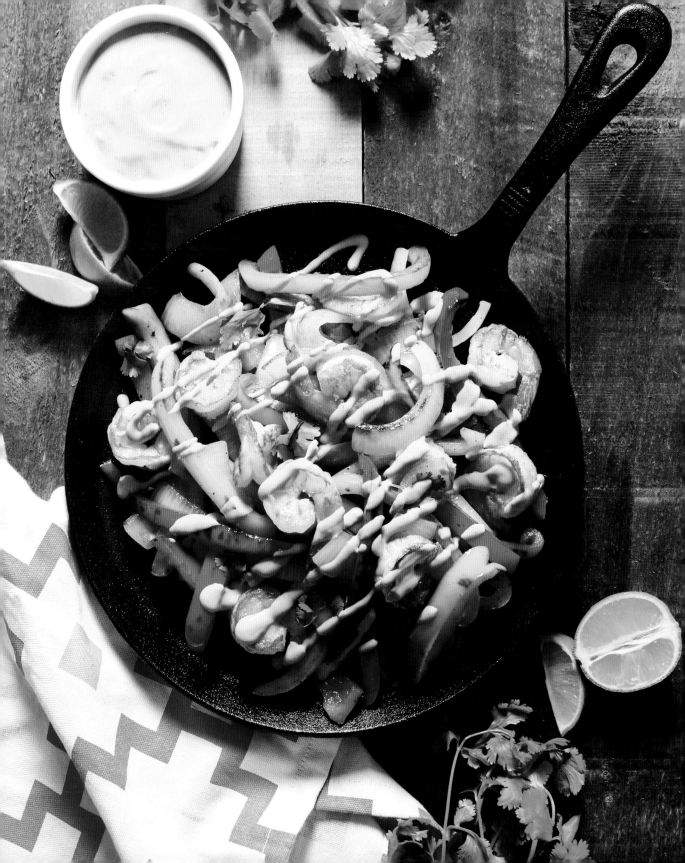

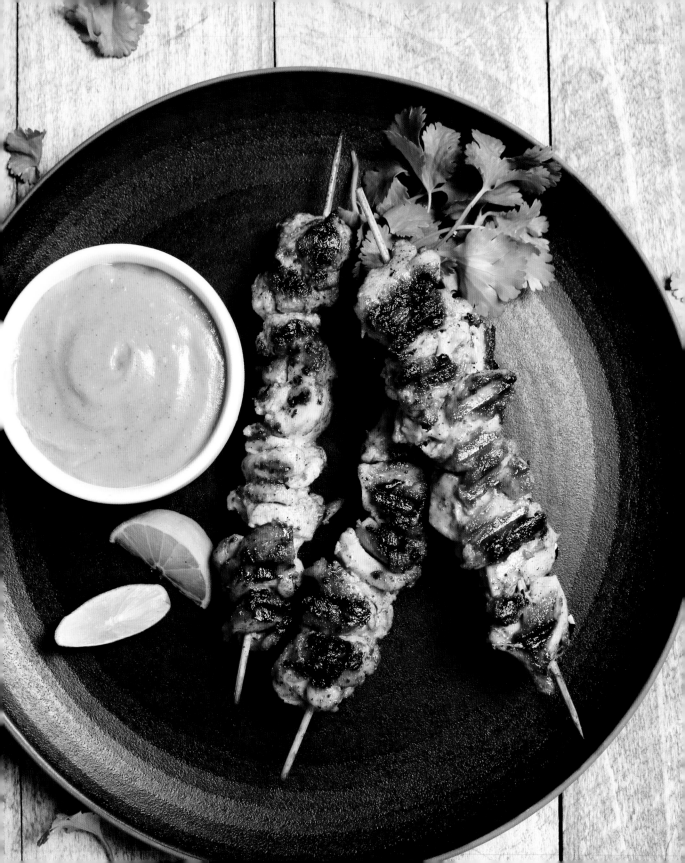

CHICKEN SATAY

1½ lb (680 g) boneless, skinless chicken thighs

1 cup (225 g) coconut cream

2 tbsp (13 g) curry powder

Juice of ½ lime

1 tsp kosher salt

EASY PEANUT SAUCE

1 cup (225 g) coconut cream

⅓ cup (87 g) natural, no-sugar-added, smooth peanut butter

1 tbsp (15 ml) soy sauce

1 tbsp (12 g) erythritol or allulose sweetener

Lime wedges or fresh cilantro leaves, for garnish

MACROS *per* SERVING

Calories: 784 • Fat: 54.4 g

Carbs: 8.7 g • Net Carbs: 7.2 g

Protein: 51.1 g

BANGKOK CHICKEN SATAY WITH PEANUT SAUCE

There was a giant open-air restaurant next to a temple in the middle of Bangkok that specialized in chicken satay. That's all the restaurant makes, and they absolutely perfected it. This recipe is a re-creation of that perfect meal from the streets of Thailand. The chicken is smoky and complex from the subtle curry notes, while the sauce is creamy and sweet.

Have six to eight skewers ready. If they are wooden, start by soaking them in water.

Marinate the chicken: Slice the chicken thighs into 1-inch (2.5-cm) cubes. Place them in a bowl along with the coconut cream, curry powder and lime juice. Mix to combine everything and let marinate for at least 15 minutes.

Meanwhile, prepare the peanut sauce: In a small saucepan, combine all the sauce ingredients. Slowly warm over medium-low heat, stirring constantly, until the sauce comes together. Do not boil it. Turn off the heat once the sauce is smooth and creamy.

Thread the meat, tightly packing it, onto the skewers. Shake off the excess marinade, then sprinkle the skewers evenly with the teaspoon of salt. You can cook the skewers on an outdoor grill, on a cast-iron grill pan or even on a cookie sheet, using the broil function of your oven. Grill the skewers over high heat for about 10 minutes, flipping over halfway through. You want to make sure you char the edges, to get some color and smoky flavor. If you're using a cookie sheet under the broiler, place the cookie sheet on the oven's top rack and cook the skewers until they are charred. Flip them over, and repeat on the other side.

Serve the skewers with a side of the peanut sauce and garnish with lime wedges or cilantro leaves.

1 lb (455 g) ground lamb

2 tsp (12 g) kosher salt

2 tsp (5 g) paprika

½ tsp ground cinnamon

1 tsp freshly ground black pepper

2 tsp (6 g) garlic powder

⅛ tsp cayenne pepper (optional)

1 large egg

1 tbsp (15 ml) olive oil

1 batch Easy Tahini Yogurt Sauce (page 149)

MACROS *per* SERVING

Calories: 473 • Fat: 40.1 g

Carbs: 2.1 g • Net Carbs: 1.9 g

Protein: 16.8 g

SPICED LAMB MEATBALLS

This recipe is a great way to introduce more lamb into your diet. These meatballs will surprise you with how simple they are to make, and you won't need the bread crumbs to keep these meatballs moist and tender. The warm spices pair perfectly with the lamb. If you want a way to reinvigorate your lunch menu, this recipe will definitely deliver.

Preheat your oven to 450°F (230°C). Line a baking sheet with aluminum foil.

In a large bowl, combine the lamb with the salt, paprika, cinnamon, black pepper, garlic powder, cayenne (if using) and the egg. Using rubber gloves for easy cleanup, mix well, using your hands. Roll the mixture into equal-sized meatballs—I like to use a 2-inch (5-cm) ice-cream scoop to form perfectly equal meatballs—and place the meatballs on a plate.

Spread the olive oil on the prepared baking sheet. Place the meatballs on the pan and roll them in the olive oil to completely coat them in oil. Spread them in an even layer and bake for 15 minutes or until just cooked through and firm. Once done, serve them with the tahini yogurt sauce.

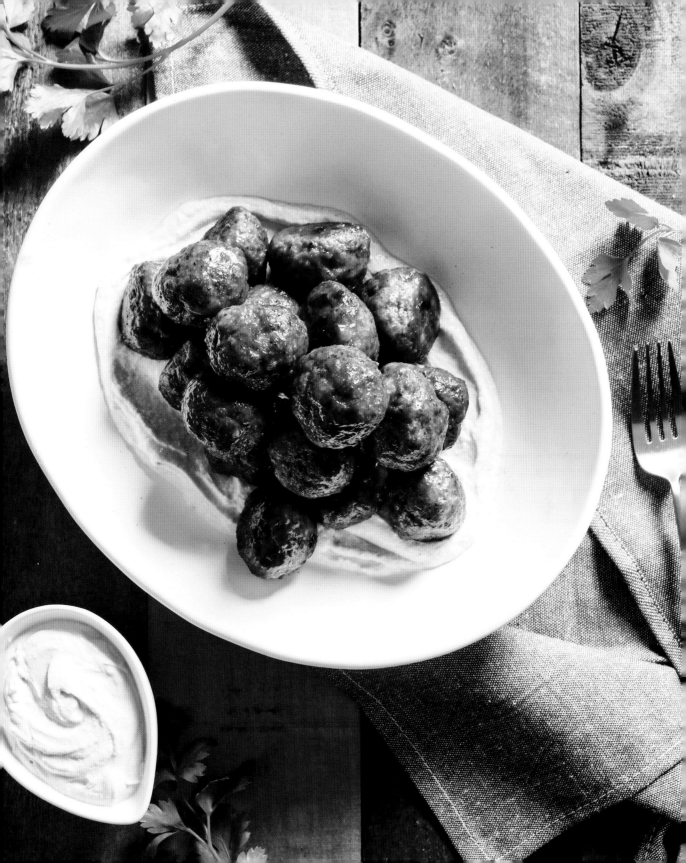

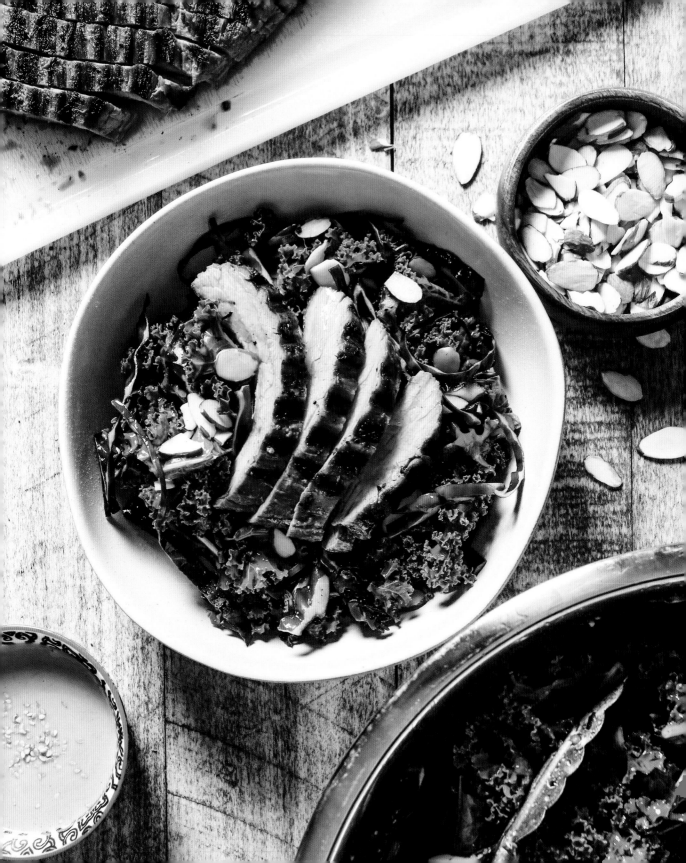

SERVES 4

1 lb (455 g) flank steak

1 batch Japanese Sesame Ginger Dressing (page 150), divided

½ head red cabbage (about 1 lb [455 g])

6 oz (170 g) chopped kale (buy the bags of precleaned and chopped kale)

¼ cup (28 g) sliced almonds

Avocado slices (optional)

MACROS *per* SERVING

Calories: 463 • Fat: 32.1 g

Carbs: 13.8 g • Net Carbs: 9.6 g

Protein: 30.7 g

HEARTY GRILLED STEAK & KALE SALAD

This salad is big, hearty and beautiful and is packed with unexpected ingredients and flavors that will fill you up and leave you nourished. The steak, marinated in Japanese Sesame Ginger Dressing (page 150), is so juicy and flavorful, you'll want to eat it on its own. But once it's added to this crunchy salad, you'll truly fall in love.

First, place the flank steak in a large bowl or a gallon-sized (4-L) ziplock bag. Add half of the ginger dressing and marinate the steak for at least 30 minutes, or up to 12 hours.

Meanwhile, remove the thick part of the core/stem from the half cabbage. Then, shave the cabbage, as you would for slaw, into thin strips. In a large bowl, combine the cabbage and kale with the remaining ginger dressing. Using tongs (or your hands), gently mix and massage the dressing into the salad for 2 to 3 minutes, which will soften the kale. Then, add the almonds and give it all a final mix. Place the salad in the fridge.

Get your grill or cast-iron grill pan piping hot. Place your flank steak on the grill and grill on high for 4 to 5 minutes, or until dark grill marks are visible. Flip over to the other side and grill for another 4 minutes (for medium-rare steak). If you prefer your steak cooked to medium, cook for 6 minutes on each side. Once done, let it rest on a cutting board for 10 minutes. Then, slice it against the grain.

Transfer the salad to four wide bowls, then top it with a few slices of steak on each. Add sliced avocado (if using).

QUICK-PICKLED VEGGIES

5½ oz (150 g) daikon

1 cup (240 ml) white vinegar

1 cup (240 ml) water

½ cup (98 g) erythritol or allulose sweetener

3 oz (80 g) precut carrot matchsticks

SEASONED PORK

2 tbsp (28 g) coconut oil

4 cloves garlic

1 lb (455 g) ground pork

2 tbsp (30 ml) soy sauce

1 tsp Asian fish sauce

1 tbsp (12 g) erythritol or allulose sweetener

1 tsp freshly ground black pepper

TO ASSEMBLE

1 head Bibb or butter lettuce, leaves separated

½ cup (115 g) mayonnaise

½ cup packed (25 g) fresh cilantro

Sriracha sauce, for drizzling (optional)

MACROS *per* SERVING

Calories: 805 • Fat: 67.2 g

Carbs: 7.9 g • Net Carbs: 6 g

Protein: 40.7 g

VIETNAMESE "BANH MI" LETTUCE WRAPS

This Keto version of the classic Vietnamese sandwich makes for a fun and funky twist on lunch. You won't be missing the baguette once you try the sweet and salty perfection of the quick-pickled veggies and savory meat. Just don't forget lots of fresh cilantro and mayo to complete the perfect bite! Save any leftover pickled veggies in the fridge for a tasty snack.

Make the pickled vegetables: Julienne-cut the daikon into small "matchsticks" by first cutting the top and bottom off of the daikon, leaving one 2-inch (5-cm) segment. Then, cut off four sides to create a peeled rectangular shape. Cut into very thin slices about ⅛ inch (3 mm) thick, then lay the slices flat and cut evenly into matchsticks. Meanwhile, in a small saucepan, bring the vinegar, water and sweetener to a boil. Once boiling, drop in the carrot matchsticks and daikon. Immediately turn off the heat and let the veggies rest in the warm vinegar mixture for at least 10 minutes.

Prepare the pork: Place a large, nonstick skillet over high heat. Add the coconut oil, garlic and ground pork. Break up the meat and sauté for 1 minute, and then add the soy sauce, fish sauce, sweetener and pepper. Sauté just until the meat is cooked, about 4 minutes.

Assemble the wraps: Generously coat the inside of each lettuce leaf with mayo, then add a scoop of cooked meat, then pickled veggies and finally a nice amount of fresh cilantro. If you like it spicy, I recommend adding a drizzle of sriracha on top. Yum!

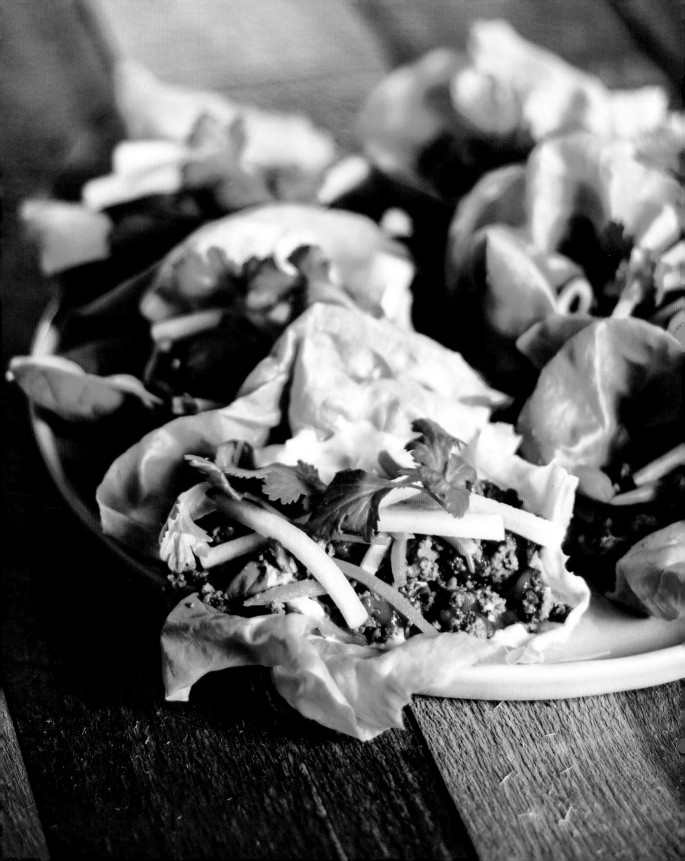

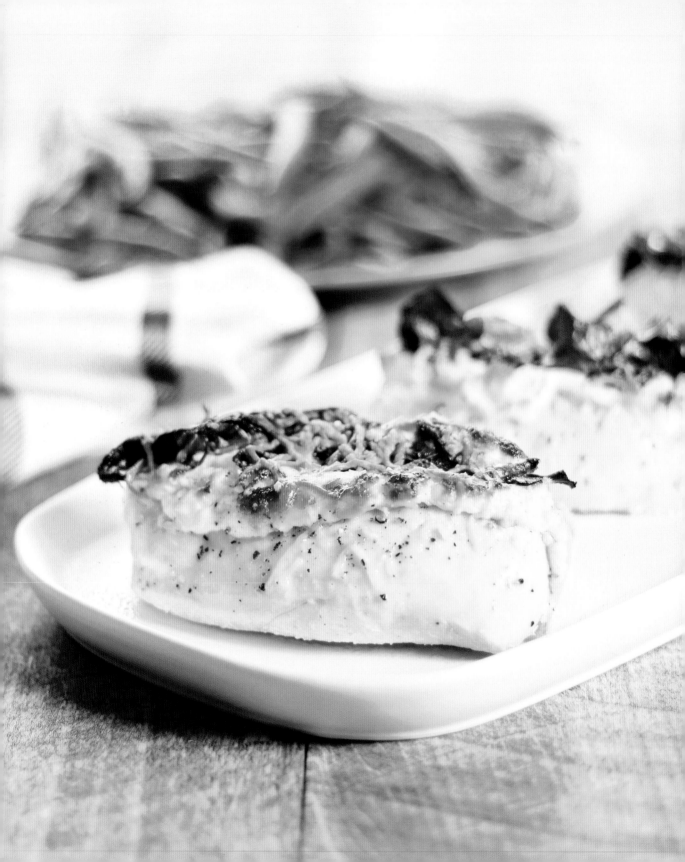

2 lb (905 g) boneless, skinless chicken breast (3 pieces)

2 tbsp (30 ml) olive oil

¼ tsp kosher salt

¼ tsp freshly ground black pepper

5.2 oz (150 g) Boursin "Garlic & Fine Herbs" cheese

1 cup (35 g) fresh spinach

¼ cup (20 g) shredded Parmesan cheese

1 batch Meyer Lemon Vinaigrette (page 146; optional)

MACROS *per* SERVING

Calories: 775   •   Fat: 37 g

Carbs: 3.8 g   •   Net Carbs: 3.5 g

Protein: 100.8 g

BOURSIN-STUFFED CHICKEN

Boursin cheese, the garlic and herb spread, is one of those treats I remember first tasting as a kid. I still remember spreading it on crackers and being positively mind-blown. But using it to stuff chicken just takes it to new heights. This dish could not be easier, and it is absolutely decadent and delicious. Stuffing the chicken with the creamy cheese really helps keep the white meat moist and tender. And if you want to turn this into a nice dinner, serve it with a batch of the Perfect Mashed "Faux-tatoes" (page 101).

Leave the chicken out of the fridge for 30 minutes prior to cooking. Meanwhile, preheat your oven to 375°F (190°C). Line a rimmed baking sheet with aluminum foil for easy cleanup.

Using a sharp knife, cut a slit from the top, straight down, to about halfway to the bottom of the meat (do not slice all the way through the chicken). Place the chicken breasts on the prepared pan and coat all sides of the chicken with the olive oil. Sprinkle the chicken evenly on all sides with the salt and pepper.

Divide the Boursin into equal thirds and press one-third into the opening of each piece of chicken. Next, divide the spinach leaves into thirds and press the spinach leaves into the Boursin. Finally, sprinkle the tops with the shredded Parmesan. Bake on the center rack of the oven for 35 to 40 minutes, or until the chicken has an internal temperature of 165°F (73°C). Serve it on a platter with a drizzle of the Meyer lemon vinaigrette (if using).

Inspired
WEEKNIGHT
MEALS

EVEN ON A WEEKNIGHT YOU CAN GET A DELICIOUS, exciting meal on the table for your family. These meals have big flavors without the carbs or the big budget. With many one-pot or sheet pan meals in this chapter, you'll be sure to find something easy and quick enough to add to your weekly dinner menu.

Rosemary Dijon Chicken & Haricots Verts (page 40)

Mediterranean Roasted Salmon & Brussels Sprouts (page 43)

Seared Ribeye with Blue Cheese & Chive Compound Butter (page 44)

Lemon Caper Shrimp & Avocado (page 47)

Miso-Glazed Pork Ribs (page 48)

Juicy Argentinean Skirt Steak & Chimichurri (page 51)

The Chicken-Bacon-Mushroom Skillet (page 52)

Slow Cooker Carnitas with Ancho Chile (page 55)

Salmon Croquettes with Turmeric-Ginger Aioli (page 56)

Creamy Sun-Dried Tomato Chicken (page 59)

Grilled Chicken Shawarma with Dill Yogurt Sauce (page 60)

Pork Chops with Creamy Mushroom Sauce (page 63)

Korean BBQ Pork Belly (page 64)

Instant Pot Paneer Korma (page 67)

2 lb (905 g) large, bone-in, skin-on chicken thighs

2 tsp (12 g) kosher salt, divided

1 tsp freshly ground black pepper, divided

2 tbsp (30 ml) avocado oil

¼ cup (57 g or ½ stick) unsalted butter

4 cloves garlic, finely chopped

¼ cup (88 g) Dijon mustard

1½ tsp (2 g) dried rosemary

1 cup (240 ml) heavy whipping cream (or coconut cream for dairy-free)

1 (1-lb [455-g]) bag fresh haricots verts (a.k.a. French beans)

MACROS *per* SERVING

Calories: 911 • Fat: 74.7 g

Carbs: 9.5 g • Net Carbs: 6.7 g

Protein: 40.9 g

ROSEMARY DIJON CHICKEN & HARICOTS VERTS

This one-pot meal is just fancy enough to impress, but cheap and easy enough for any weeknight dinner at home. Packed with flavor, this is the juiciest chicken you'll ever have—a definite winner-winner chicken dinner!

Preheat your oven to 425°F (220°C). Remove the chicken thighs from the package and place them on a plate. Pat the skin dry with a paper towel and evenly coat both sides with 1 teaspoon of the salt and ½ teaspoon of the pepper.

Place a large skillet over medium-high heat. Add the oil and heat until the oil starts to smoke. Place the chicken, skin side down, in the pan. Leave it, without touching it, for exactly 5 minutes, to form a crispy skin. You want a nice, dark brown color on the skin. Turn it over and sear the bottom for 2 minutes. Turn off the heat and remove the chicken, placing it on a plate. (Caution: The chicken is not fully cooked. This step was just to brown the skin.)

While the pan is still hot, add the butter and garlic. As the butter melts, use a spatula to stir and scrape the fond off the bottom of the pan. Then, stir in the mustard, rosemary, cream and remaining teaspoon of salt and ½ teaspoon of pepper. Add the haricots verts and toss them with your tongs to combine. Arrange the chicken thighs on top of the haricots verts, with the chicken skin side up. Just make sure the chicken skin is not submerged in the sauce, as we want that skin to remain crispy. Bake everything for 20 minutes, or until the chicken has an internal temperature of 165°F (73°C). Serve family style right in the skillet, and dig in!

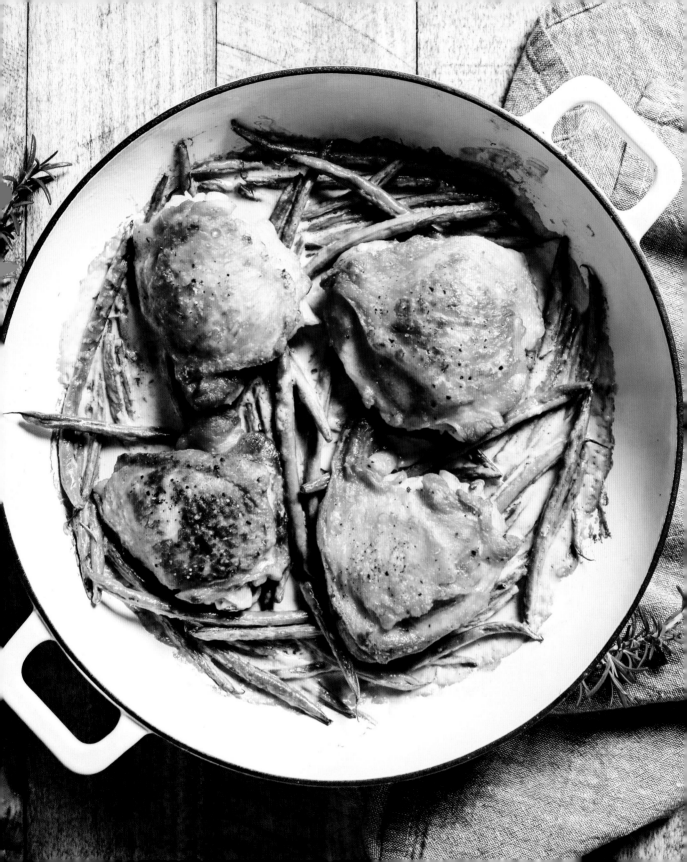

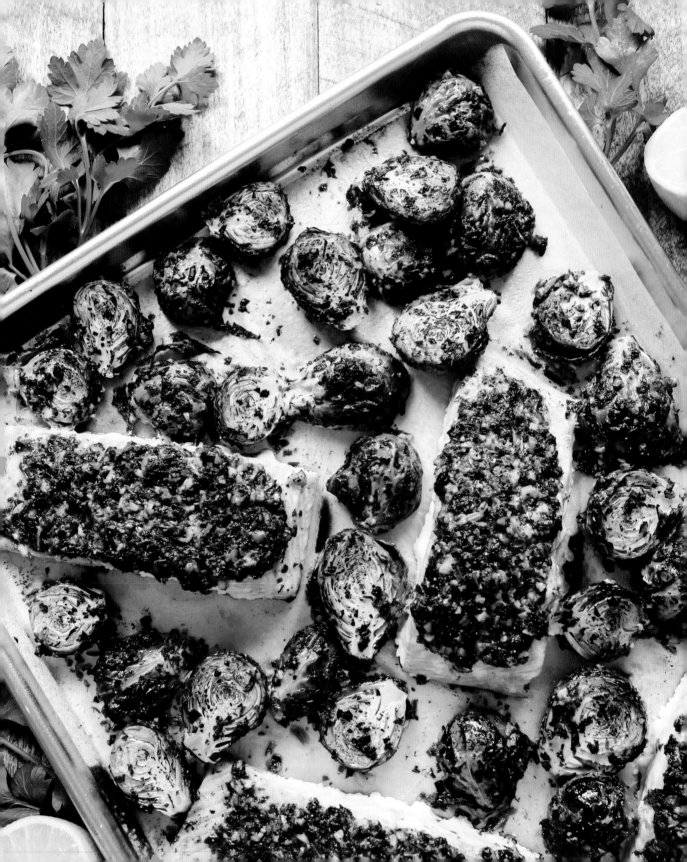

SERVES 4

Olive oil, for baking sheet

1 lb (455 g) Brussels sprouts

8 cloves garlic

1 bunch parsley (2½ oz [70 g]),
stems removed

1 tbsp (18 g) kosher salt

2 tsp (4 g) freshly ground black
pepper

2 tsp (2 g) dried dill, or ¼ oz (7 g) fresh,
chopped

Juice of 2 lemons

½ cup (120 ml) olive oil

4 (6-oz [170-g]) skin-on salmon fillets
(1½ lb [680 g] total)

Lemon slices or fresh parsley,
for garnish

MACROS *per* SERVING

Calories: 600 • Fat: 46.8 g

Carbs: 11.2 g • Net Carbs: 7.3 g

Protein: 33.8 g

MEDITERRANEAN ROASTED SALMON & BRUSSELS SPROUTS

This bright and sunny dinner is loaded with lemon and herbs for a fresh take on roasted salmon. The Mediterranean flavors really pack a punch, and this beautiful dish is full of healthy fats and nutrients. The best part is, it's a sheet pan meal that you just toss in the oven. Easy enough for any day of the week.

Try pairing this with the Garlic Aioli (page 141).

Preheat your oven to 475°F (240°C). Line a baking sheet with aluminum foil for easy cleanup, then grease the foil with a little bit of olive oil. Slice the Brussels sprouts in half and set them aside in a large mixing bowl.

In a food processor, blend the garlic, parsley, salt, pepper, dill, lemon juice and olive oil to make an herb rub.

Place the 4 salmon fillets, skin side down, on the prepared baking sheet. Scoop a heaping spoonful of herb rub and spread it on top of each fillet. Add the rest of the rub to the Brussels sprouts and stir to combine. Evenly spread the Brussels sprouts around the fillets. Bake on the top rack of the oven for 15 minutes, then turn the oven to broil and broil for another 5 minutes, or until the Brussels sprouts have a nice crispy exterior.

Serve family style right out of the baking sheet, or plate the salmon with a side of Brussels sprouts for each person. Garnish with a slice of lemon or some fresh parsley.

BLUE CHEESE & CHIVE COMPOUND BUTTER

¼ cup (57 g or ½ stick) salted butter, at room temperature (not melted)

¼ cup (32 g) crumbled blue cheese

1 tbsp (4 g) finely chopped fresh chives

SEARED RIBEYE

2 (1-lb [455-g]) ribeye steaks, 1" (2.5 cm) thick

1 tsp kosher salt

½ tsp freshly ground black pepper

¼ cup (57 g or ½ stick) unsalted butter

3 cloves garlic

1 rosemary sprig

MACROS *per* SERVING

Calories: 687 • Fat: 47.4 g

Carbs: 0.7 g • Net Carbs: 0.7 g

Protein: 67.4 g

SEARED RIBEYE WITH BLUE CHEESE & CHIVE COMPOUND BUTTER

This recipe walks you through, step-by-step, how to sear the perfect ribeye like a chef. The compound butter elevates this rustic dish to steak house quality and will have you licking the plate clean. The creamy blue cheese combines perfectly with the butter and the delicate onion flavor from the chives. Even those who don't like blue cheese will love this. Try pairing this with the Cheesy Brussels Sprout Gratin (page 102).

Prepare the compound butter: In a food processor, blend the butter on high speed until it's fluffy. Then, add the blue cheese and chives. Continue to blend until the mixture is totally smooth. Lay a sheet of plastic wrap on your counter. Remove the compound butter from the processor and place it in the center of the plastic wrap. Gently roll up the butter in the plastic wrap, forming a cylinder. Twist the ends of the plastic wrap to seal the butter. Place it in the fridge to chill.

Prepare the ribeye: Remove the steaks from your fridge at least 15 minutes before cooking. Pat the steaks dry with a paper towel. Then, coat them evenly with salt and pepper. Use ¼ teaspoon of salt and ⅛ teaspoon of pepper on each side of each steak.

Place a large, cast-iron skillet over high heat without oil. Once it's smoking hot, place your steaks in the pan. Cook, without touching the steaks, for exactly 4 minutes. Flip them over and cook for 3 minutes. Then, add the butter, garlic and rosemary. Using an oven mitt, if needed, hold the pan at an angle so the butter pools, and use a soup spoon to baste the steak with the butter for 2 minutes. Remove the steaks and place them on a cutting board to rest for exactly 5 minutes. You can slice off and discard any large pieces of fat around the edges and then slice the meat into ¼-inch (6-mm) strips.

To serve, top with a generous pat of the compound butter.

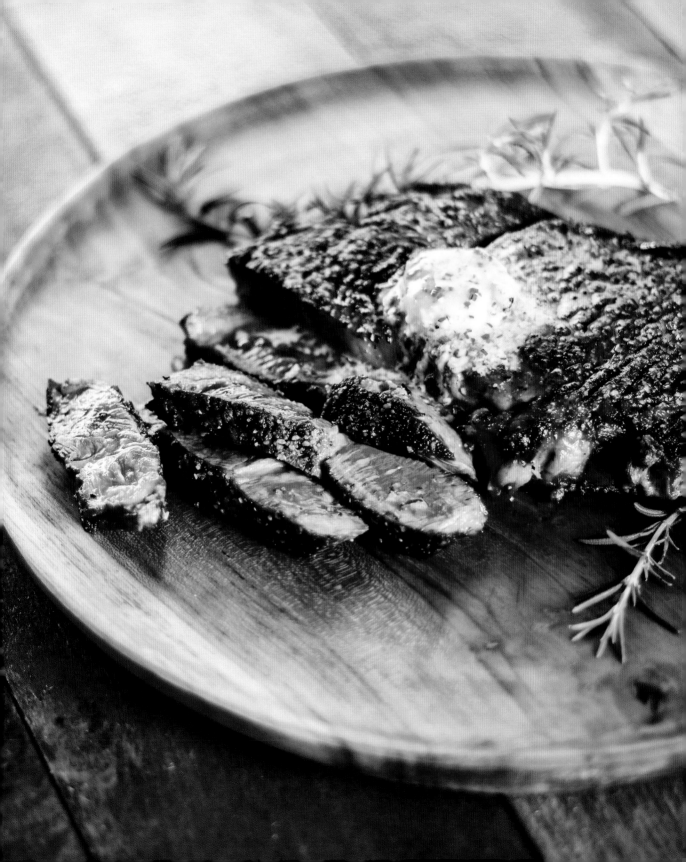

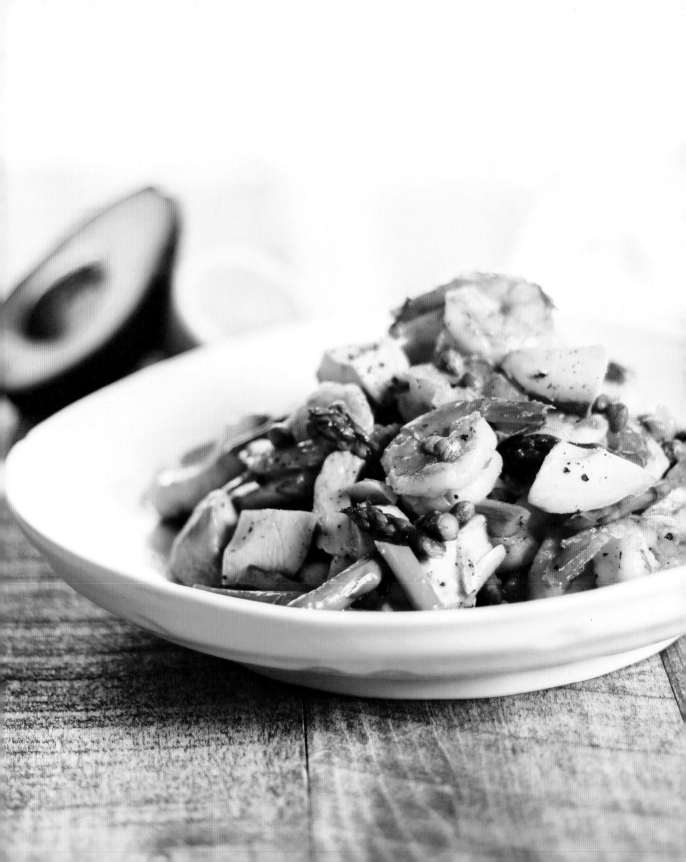

½ cup (112 g or 1 stick) unsalted butter

8 cloves garlic, thinly sliced

2 lb (905 g) shrimp (21–30 count), thawed, peeled and deveined

1 lb (455 g) asparagus, sliced into 1" (2.5-cm) pieces

2 tsp (12 g) kosher salt

½ tsp freshly ground black pepper, plus more for garnish

Juice of 1 lemon

2 tbsp (17 g) capers

1 tbsp (15 ml) caper juice from jar

2 avocados, peeled, pitted and cubed

MACROS *per* SERVING

Calories: 496 • Fat: 35.2 g

Carbs: 12.4 g • Net Carbs: 5.7 g

Protein: 34.7 g

LEMON CAPER SHRIMP & AVOCADO

This is one of our household weeknight staples. The recipe is so quick and easy and just exploding with flavor. Packed with healthy fats, this really is the perfect Keto meal. The creamy avocado perfectly contrasts with the zesty lemon and salty capers. And the brown butter and shrimp are just the right kind of sweet.

In a large, cast-iron or nonstick skillet over high heat, combine the butter and garlic. Once the butter is melted and bubbly, add the shrimp, sliced asparagus, salt and pepper. Sauté for 1 minute. Then, add the lemon juice, capers and caper juice. Sauté for 1 more minute, stirring constantly.

Immediately remove the pan from the heat and add the avocado cubes, then toss everything together very gently as the avocado is fragile. Pour the mixture into a serving bowl and top it with freshly cracked black pepper.

MISO-GLAZED PORK RIBS

PRESSURE COOKER RIBS

1 (3-lb [1.4-kg]) rack baby back ribs

½ cup (125 g) red miso paste

½ cup (120 ml) Shaoxing wine or sake

1 tbsp (15 ml) low-sodium soy sauce

1 tbsp (15 ml) cider vinegar (I prefer Bragg organic)

MISO GLAZE

½ cup (120 ml) Shaoxing wine or sake

½ cup (125 g) red miso paste

⅔ cup (130 g) allulose sweetener

½ tsp freshly ground black pepper

TO SERVE

3 scallions, thinly sliced into rings

Sesame seeds, for garnish (optional)

MACROS *per* SERVING

Calories: 831 • Fat: 54 g

Carbs: 9.1 g • Net Carbs: 9.1 g

Protein: 67.5 g

Now that I'm living in Texas, ribs have become a big part of my daily life. Tender, juicy, messy ribs are truly a one-of-a-kind treat. But this recipe adds a twist by using Japanese miso paste to bring a powerful hit of umami to the party. These ribs are truly finger-lickin' good. And the sweet and salty miso glaze is packed with flavor (and healthy probiotics) that make this recipe special. The best part is that you don't need all day to make these ribs, since we'll use a pressure cooker or Instant Pot®.

Try pairing this with Jicama & Orange Slaw (page 113).

Prepare the ribs: Remove the membrane from the back (bone side) of the rack of ribs. Use a paper towel to grip the slippery membrane and pull it off. Cut the rack into three equal parts, roughly 6 inches (15 cm) in length.

Coat all sides of the ribs in the miso paste. In the pressure cooker or Instant Pot, combine the Shaoxing wine, soy sauce and cider vinegar. Then, add the ribs, standing them upright on the bones. Cook the ribs on high pressure for 25 minutes.

While the ribs cook, make the glaze: In a small saucepan, combine the Shaoxing wine, miso paste, allulose and pepper. Over medium heat, bring the sauce to a boil and simmer for a minute or two, whisking constantly, just until everything dissolves and the glaze becomes thick and syrupy.

To finish the dish, turn your oven to broil and line a baking sheet with aluminum foil. Release the pressure from the pressure cooker and very carefully transfer the ribs to the prepared baking sheet. Use a silicone brush to generously coat all sides of the ribs with the glaze. Place the ribs on the top rack of the oven and broil them for 3 to 4 minutes, or until the top starts to caramelize. Remove them from the oven and brush on another layer of glaze on the top of the ribs.

To serve, top with the sliced scallions and a sprinkle of sesame seeds (if using).

PRO TIP: If you have a smoker at home, try smoking the ribs for 4 hours at 225°F (107°C) wrapped in aluminum foil, then finishing under the broiler with the glaze.

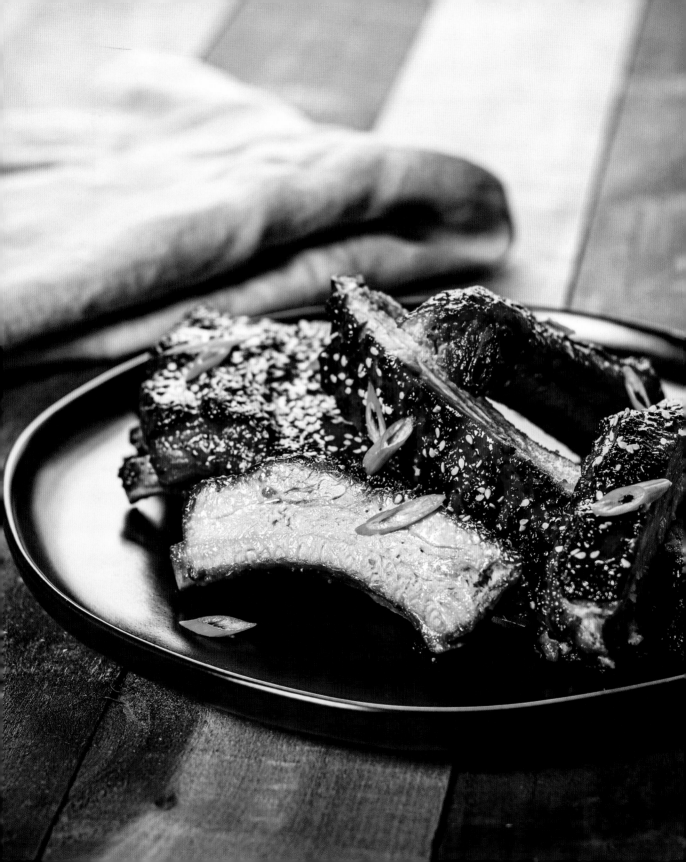

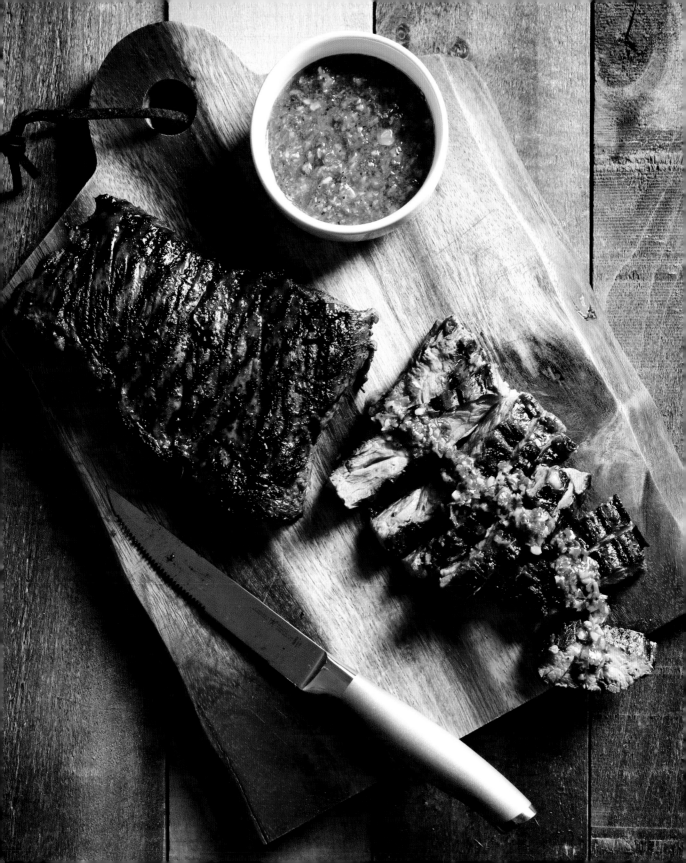

MARINATED SKIRT STEAK

1½ lb (680 g) skirt steak

2 tbsp (30 ml) low-sodium soy sauce

3 tbsp (45 ml) Worcestershire sauce

Juice of ½ lemon

½ tsp freshly ground black pepper

CLASSIC CHIMICHURRI

⅓ cup (80 ml) olive oil

1 cup firmly packed (65 g) fresh parsley, stems removed

6 cloves garlic

Juice of ½ lemon

2 tbsp (30 ml) cider vinegar (I prefer Bragg organic)

1 tsp kosher salt

½ tsp freshly ground black pepper

MACROS *per* SERVING

Calories: 869 • Fat: 67.4 g

Carbs: 3.6 g • Net Carbs: 2.9 g

Protein: 63.6 g

JUICY ARGENTINEAN SKIRT STEAK & CHIMICHURRI

This recipe will definitely bring you right to South America. The marriage of the zesty chimichurri with the marinated skirt steak makes this a dinner your family will be begging you to cook again. Marinating the skirt steak makes an inexpensive cut of beef juicy and tender. And the process is surprisingly easy.

Try pairing this with the Button Mushroom Flambé (page 110).

Prepare the skirt steak: Carefully trim off any large/thick pieces of fat or silver skin on the surface. It doesn't need to be perfect, but any thick fat will become chewy. Cut the skirt steak in half into two equal-sized pieces.

In a large bowl or gallon-sized (4-L) ziplock bag, combine the soy sauce, Worcestershire, lemon juice and pepper. Stir, then add the steak. Let the steak marinate for at least 30 minutes, or up to 4 hours.

Make the chimichurri: In a food processor, combine all the chimichurri ingredients and blend until the mixture is smooth.

When ready to cook the steak, bring a cast-iron grill pan or your outdoor grill to high heat. Once smoking hot, add the steak and grill it for 4 to 5 minutes, or until a dark brown crust has formed. Flip it once and cook for another 4 minutes. Place the steak on a cutting board and let it rest for at least 10 minutes. Then, slice it, against the grain, into ¼-inch (6-mm) slices. Drizzle the chimichurri over the top and serve.

PRO TIP: For an extra twist, use the Spicy Red Chimichurri (page 138) instead of the classic version here.

8 oz (225 g) no-sugar-added bacon

2 lb (905 g) thinly sliced boneless, skinless chicken breast

1 tsp kosher salt

½ tsp freshly ground black pepper

1 lb (455 g) cremini mushrooms, cleaned

5 cloves garlic, finely chopped

1 cup (240 ml) low-sodium beef stock

1 tbsp (15 ml) soy sauce

1 tbsp (15 ml) Worcestershire sauce

½ cup (55 g) shredded Gruyère or Swiss cheese

Chopped fresh parsley, for garnish (optional)

MACROS *per* SERVING

Calories: 575 • Fat: 27.2 g

Carbs: 6.8 g • Net Carbs: 5.6 g

Protein: 76.8 g

THE CHICKEN-BACON-MUSHROOM SKILLET

Doesn't the name say it all? Pretty much all the best things in one pot! This dish is packed with savory goodness and fits perfectly into the Keto lifestyle. The chicken, bacon and mushrooms come together to create the most incredible sauce, and it's all covered in gooey cheese. This is one of my weeknight go-tos, as it is comforting, easy to make and totally delicious.

Preheat your oven to broil. While the oven heats, slice the bacon into ½-inch (1.3-cm) pieces and season both sides of the chicken with salt and pepper. Then, heat a large cast-iron or ovenproof nonstick skillet over high heat. Fry the bacon pieces for about 4 minutes, or until crispy. Remove the bacon from the pan and set aside, but leave the grease in the pan.

Add the chicken to the pan and sear it for 2 minutes on each side, or until both sides have been browned (you may need to do this in two batches). Transfer the chicken to a plate.

Add the mushrooms and garlic to the pan, and sauté for 1 minute. Add the stock, soy sauce and Worcestershire, and stir to combine, scraping the fond off the bottom of the pan.

Add the chicken back to the pan, submerging it slightly in the sauce. Bring everything to a boil, then top with the bacon and sprinkle with the shredded cheese. Place the skillet under the broiler until the cheese gets bubbly. Garnish with chopped parsley (if using) and serve it up family style.

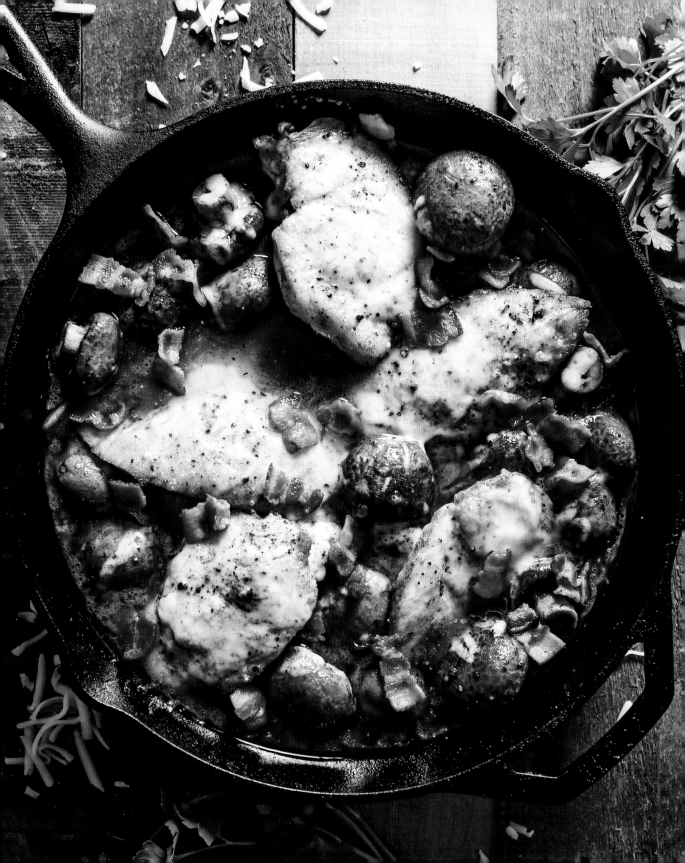

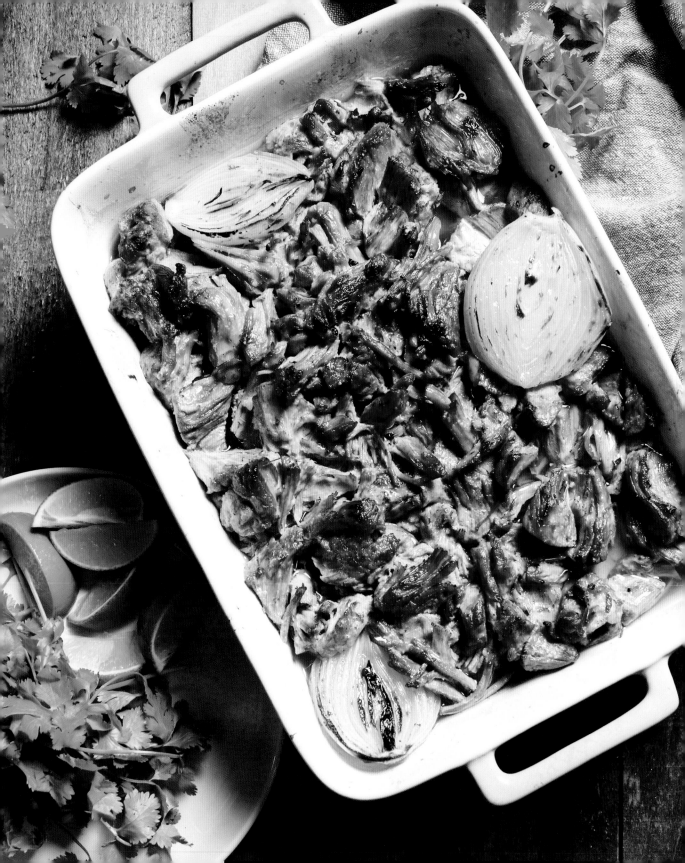

1 (3½-lb [1.6-kg]) pork butt/shoulder

2 large white onions

1 bunch cilantro

32 oz (946 ml) low-sodium chicken stock

2 tbsp (30 ml) cider vinegar (I prefer Bragg organic)

3 bay leaves

1¼ oz (35 g) dried ancho chiles (3 or 4 whole chiles)

2 tbsp (36 g) kosher salt

1 tsp freshly ground black pepper

Low-carb tortillas, lettuce, cheese, sour cream, salsa or avocado slices, for serving

MACROS *per* SERVING

Calories: 617 • Fat: 42.8 g

Carbs: 1.3 g • Net Carbs: 1.1 g

Protein: 52.8 g

SLOW COOKER CARNITAS WITH ANCHO CHILE

Traditional carnitas in Mexico involves cooking pork in its own fat, and that's exactly what is going to happen in this recipe. Using a slow cooker makes this super easy and yields the juiciest, tenderest meat. And the dried ancho chile brings a complexity and subtle smokiness to this dish. Get ready for the most delicious, luxurious carnitas you've ever had.

Try pairing this with Avocado Salsa Verde (page 142).

Start by slicing the pork into 2-inch (5-cm) cubes and set it aside. Then, cut the onions in half, from root to tip. Carefully peel off the outer layer. Cut off the majority of the roots, but be sure to leave a tiny bit of core attached to the onion, as this will hold the onion together while it cooks. Cut off the top half of the entire bunch of cilantro (save the leafy tops for the salsa verde; we are using only the stems in this recipe). Using butcher's twine, tie a tight knot around the cilantro stems. This will make it easier to remove the stems later.

In a slow cooker or Instant Pot, combine the chicken stock, vinegar, bay leaves, dried chiles, salt and black pepper. Stir well. Then, add the pork and bundle of cilantro stems, and place the onions along the outside. Be sure everything is in an even layer. Close the lid and slow cook on high for 4 hours or low for 8 hours, or if using an Instant Pot, on the slow cook setting.

When the pork is done, use a slotted spoon to gently transfer the pork and onions to a rimmed baking sheet or cast-iron pan. Then, using a ladle, carefully transfer the fatty layer at the top of the slow cooker and pour it right over the carnitas in the pan. Make sure the liquid comes about halfway up the meat in the pan. Place the pork under your oven broiler for 5 to 10 minutes, or until the top gets brown and crispy. Serve with your favorite low-carb tortillas, or make carnitas bowls with lettuce, cheese, sour cream, salsa and avocado slices.

TURMERIC-GINGER AIOLI

½ cup (115 g) mayonnaise

¼ tsp ground turmeric

½ tsp ground ginger

½ tsp curry powder

SALMON CROQUETTES

1 lb (455 g) skinless fresh salmon

1 large egg

2 tbsp (28 g) mayonnaise

1 tbsp (11 g) Dijon mustard

1 tbsp (7 g) coconut flour

¾ tsp kosher salt

¼ tsp freshly ground black pepper

¼ cup (60 ml) avocado oil

5 oz (140 g) baby arugula (optional)

1 batch Meyer Lemon Vinaigrette (page 146; optional)

MACROS *per* SERVING

Calories: 736 • Fat: 63.7 g

Carbs: 1.7 g • Net Carbs: 1.2 g

Protein: 35.6 g

SALMON CROQUETTES WITH TURMERIC-GINGER AIOLI

This is one of the first dishes I made for my fiancé. It was our first date night at home, and the first time he tried my cooking. To this day, it's still one of his favorites. This Keto version of croquettes needs no bread crumbs at all, and you'll still get a nice crispy exterior. The unexpected aioli is lightly curried and balances perfectly with the salmon. It's also infused with lots of healthy spices, such as turmeric and ginger, which are incredibly good for you. This dish may seem simple, but it is truly a tasty treat.

Prepare the aioli: In a bowl, combine the mayo, turmeric, ginger and curry powder. Stir well, cover the bowl with plastic wrap and place it in the fridge to rest.

Prepare the croquettes: On a large cutting board, chop the salmon into a fine mince. Transfer the chopped salmon to a large bowl. Then, add the egg, mayo, mustard, coconut flour, salt and pepper. Mix well to combine.

Meanwhile, heat the oil in a large, cast-iron skillet over medium-high heat. Once it's smoking hot, use a ⅓-cup (80-ml) measuring cup to scoop the salmon mixture into separate mounds on the hot skillet, until you've used all of the salmon.

Fry the croquettes on each side for about 3 minutes, or until golden brown—you want a nice crust. Do not flatten the salmon cakes, as this will cause them to become dry. I like them to have just a little light pink in the center, so they stay moist and juicy.

When done, transfer them to a plate lined with paper towels to drain any excess oil. Serve two croquettes on a plate with a spoon-swipe of aioli and fresh arugula dressed with the vinaigrette (if using) on the side.

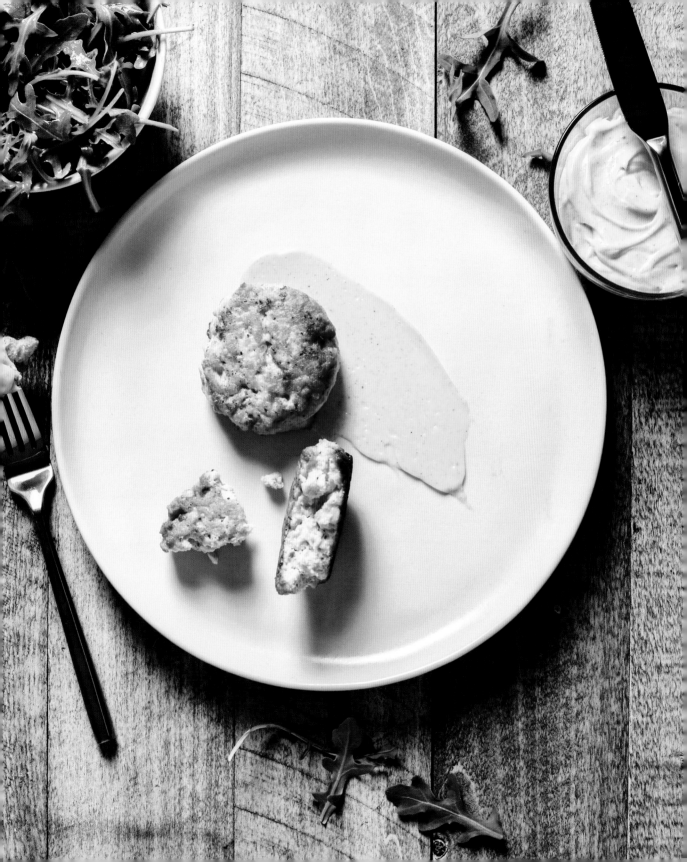

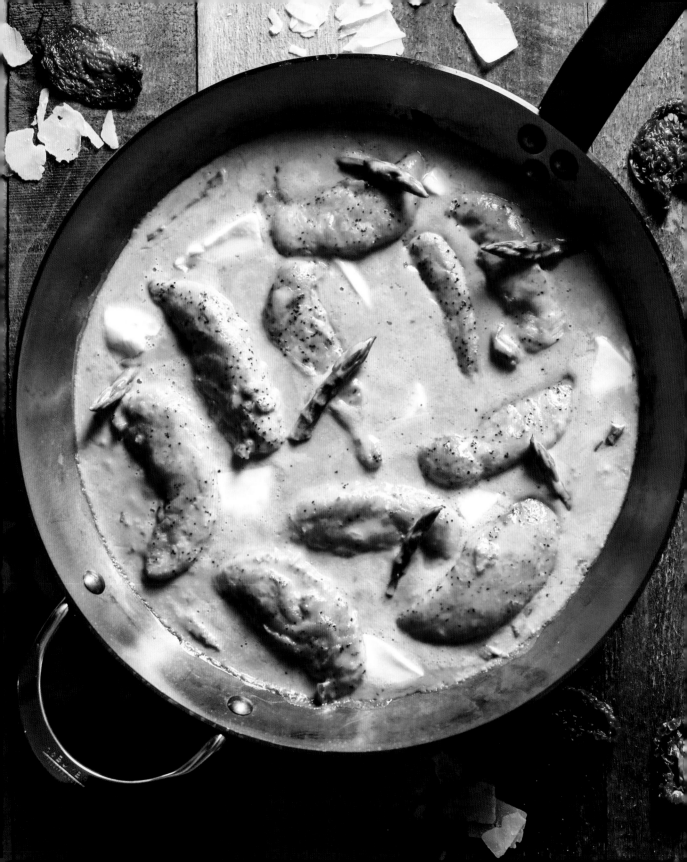

2 lb (905 g) boneless, skinless chicken breast tenders

2 tsp (6 g) garlic powder

2 tsp (12 g) kosher salt, divided

2 tbsp (30 ml) avocado oil

½ cup (120 ml) dry white wine

⅓ cup (30 g) sun-dried tomatoes, finely diced

1½ cups (355 ml) heavy whipping cream

1 cup (240 ml) low-sugar marinara sauce

½ cup (40 g) shredded Parmesan cheese, plus more for garnish

1 lb (455 g) asparagus, ends removed, sliced into 1" (2.5-cm) pieces

8 oz (225 g) fresh mozzarella cheese, cut into small pieces

Zucchini noodles or low-carb pasta (optional)

MACROS *per* SERVING

Calories: 936 • Fat: 60 g

Carbs: 5.7 g • Net Carbs: 4.2 g

Protein: 18.3 g

CREAMY SUN-DRIED TOMATO CHICKEN

Inspired by my first job working at an Italian restaurant, where I learned to make pink sauce, this one-pot dinner will have your whole family licking their plates clean. The creamy sauce is absolutely heavenly, and you'll want it by the spoonful. This recipe is also easy and quick, and will take under 30 minutes to make.

First, pat the chicken dry with a paper towel and season it on both sides with the garlic powder and 1½ teaspoons (9 g) of the salt.

Heat a large, cast-iron skillet over high heat. Add the oil, then brown both sides of the chicken just until golden brown. Remove the chicken from the pan and set it aside on a plate. (Note: The chicken may not be fully cooked.)

Lower the heat to medium and add the white wine and diced sun-dried tomatoes to the pan. As the wine cooks, scrape the bottom of the pan to remove the fond. Boil the wine for 1 to 2 minutes to cook off the alcohol, then add the cream, marinara and Parmesan, stirring well to combine. Bring the sauce back to a boil, then simmer it for 3 minutes.

Stir in the sliced asparagus, then nestle the chicken back into the sauce and simmer it for another 5 minutes. Turn off the heat and immediately top the dish with the chopped mozzarella. Sprinkle the top with extra Parmesan. Serve the finished dish family style with zucchini noodles or a low-carb pasta option (if using).

CHICKEN SHAWARMA

1½ tsp (5 g) garlic powder

½ tsp freshly ground black pepper

¼ tsp curry powder

½ tsp ground turmeric

¼ tsp ground cinnamon

2 lb (905 g) boneless, skinless chicken thighs

1½ tsp (9 g) kosher salt

YOGURT SAUCE

1 cup (230 g) full-fat, plain Greek yogurt

Juice of 1 lemon

¼ oz (7 g) fresh dill, chopped

MACROS *per* SERVING

Calories: 443 • Fat: 14.9 g

Carbs: 4.2 g • Net Carbs: 4.2 g

Protein: 65.2 g

GRILLED CHICKEN SHAWARMA WITH DILL YOGURT SAUCE

This Middle Eastern street food is one of my favorite things in the world. The unique mix of spices gives this chicken its beautiful color and flavor. The yogurt sauce is so rich and creamy and perfectly balances the zesty spices in the chicken. This recipe is a fantastic way to bring new life to chicken dinner.

Try pairing this with the Lemony Charred Broccolini (page 106).

Prepare the chicken: Preheat your oven to 350°F (180°C). Place a cast-iron grill pan over medium-high heat. In a small bowl, combine the garlic powder, pepper, curry, turmeric and cinnamon. On a cutting board, lay out the chicken thighs and evenly sprinkle the salt on both sides of the chicken. Then evenly divide the spice mixture in half and coat both sides of the chicken.

Once the grill pan is smoking hot, place the chicken, top side down, on the pan. After 5 minutes, flip the chicken. Cook for 4 minutes, then transfer the grill pan to the oven. Bake for 6 to 8 minutes, or until the chicken is fully cooked (with an internal temperature of 165°F [73°C]).

Make the sauce: In a small bowl, simply mix the yogurt with the lemon juice and chopped dill.

I like to serve this dish family style by placing the chicken on a large plate or platter with the sauce on the side in a small bowl.

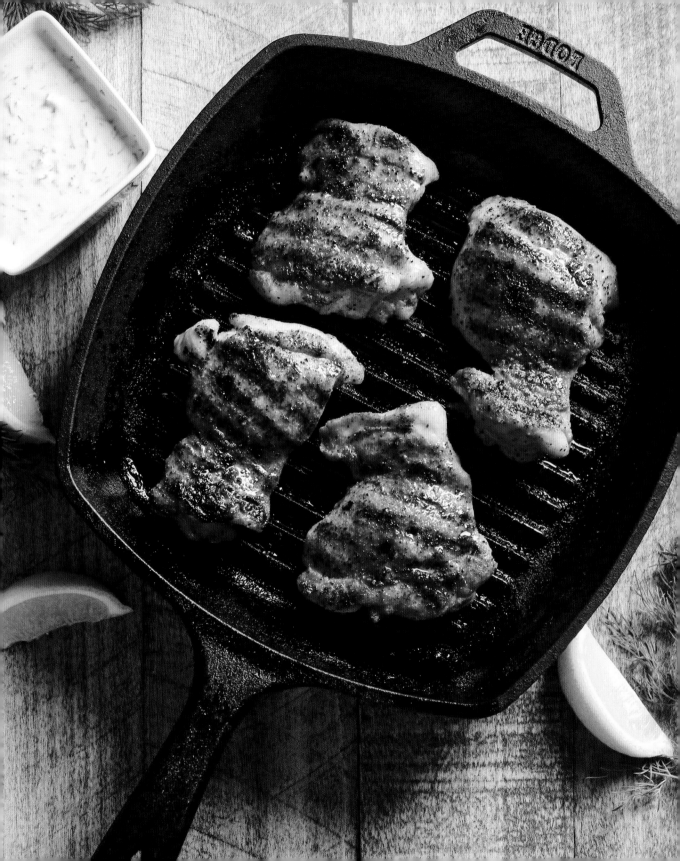

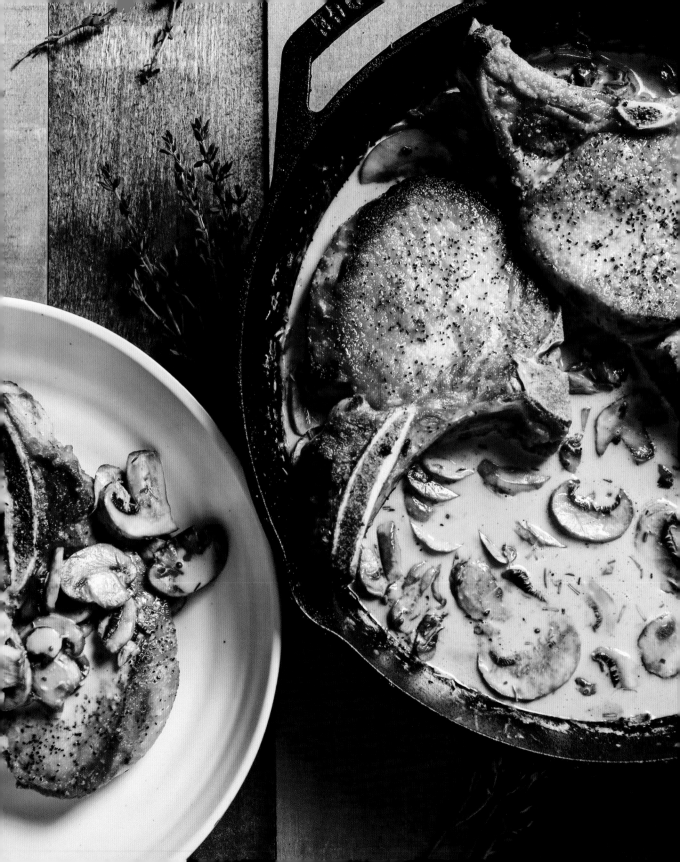

2 lb (905 g) thick-cut bone-in
pork chops

1½ lb (680 g) white mushrooms

2 tbsp (30 ml) avocado oil

1½ tsp (9 g) kosher salt, divided

1 tsp freshly ground black pepper,
divided

1 cup (240 ml) beef stock

1 cup (240 ml) heavy whipping cream
(or coconut cream for dairy-free)

4 cloves garlic, finely chopped

Leaves from 1 thyme sprig, or
½ tsp dried

2 tbsp (22 g) whole-grain mustard
(I recommend Maille "Old Style")

Extra thyme sprigs, for garnish (optional)

MACROS *per* SERVING

Calories: 831 • Fat: 55.9 g

Carbs: 7.3 g • Net Carbs: 5.8 g

Protein: 73.1 g

PORK CHOPS WITH CREAMY MUSHROOM SAUCE

This one-pot meal is a favorite at our house. The creamy mushroom sauce is absolutely decadent with the juicy pork chops and makes for the perfect easy weeknight dinner.

Let the pork rest on the counter for 20 minutes to come to room temperature. Meanwhile, slice all the mushrooms (see Pro Tip). Heat the oil in a large, cast-iron skillet over high heat. Season the pork chops with 1 teaspoon of the salt and ½ teaspoon of the pepper. Once the pan is smoking hot, add the pork chops and sear for 5 minutes. Then, flip over and sear the other side for 4 minutes. Remove the pork and set it aside on a plate to rest. (Note: The pork may not be fully cooked.)

In the hot pan still over high heat, add the stock and cream, and use a spatula to scrape the fond off the bottom of the pan. Bring the sauce to a boil and simmer for 2 to 3 minutes, then add the mushrooms, garlic, thyme, mustard and remaining ½ teaspoon each of salt and pepper. Lower the heat to medium and let the mushrooms and sauce cook for 3 more minutes. Add the pork chops on top and simmer for another 5 minutes. Serve family style, garnished with sprigs of thyme (if using).

PRO TIP: To take this recipe to the next level, try replacing some of the button mushrooms with a mix of wild mushrooms, such as chanterelle, oyster or shiitake.

KOREAN BBQ PORK BELLY

2 lb (905 g) rindless pork belly

⅓ cup (107 g) gochujang sauce,
plus more for dipping
(see Pro Tip)

½ white onion, peeled

6 cloves garlic

2 tbsp (30 ml) soy sauce

1 tbsp (15 ml) sesame oil

⅓ cup (65 g) allulose or
erythritol sweetener

1 tsp kosher salt

3 scallions, chopped into
thin rings

Sesame seeds, for garnish
(optional)

MACROS *per* SERVING

Calories: 1,279 • Fat: 123.4 g

Carbs: 16 g • Net Carbs: 13.8 g

Protein: 7.4 g

I'll never forget the tiny restaurant in Seoul that served only pork. We grilled thin slices of marinated pork belly right at the table over glowing wood embers. This recipe brings you with me back to Seoul, to put real Korean barbecue on your kitchen table. The fermented chili paste (gochujang) is the star of this dish, with its bold flavor and vibrant red color. Though traditionally made with sugar, this version of the marinade is simple to make and still packs all the sweet and salty flavors into the pork.

Remove the pork belly from the fridge and place it in the freezer to chill. In a food processor, combine the gochujang, peeled onion half, garlic, soy sauce, sesame oil, sweetener and salt. Blend on high speed for at least a full minute, until a smooth paste is formed. Set the marinade aside.

Remove the pork belly from the freezer. Cut it into long strips about 2 inches (5 cm) wide. Then, slice it into ⅛-inch (3-mm) slices. You want to work quickly, as the more you handle the pork, the more it will warm up and become more difficult to slice. Once thinly sliced, place it in a large bowl, cover it with the marinade and gently massage the pork with your hands to ensure it's covered with the marinade. Cover the bowl with plastic wrap and let it chill in the fridge for at least an hour, or overnight.

Heat up your grill outside or a cast-iron grill pan over high heat. Once it's smoking hot, grill the pork in even layers on the grill pan. You may need to do this in two batches. Cook the pork for 2 to 3 minutes on each side, until it gets nice grill marks. Once all the pork is cooked, transfer it to a large bowl and top with the sliced scallions and sesame seeds (if using). Be sure to serve a little gochujang on the side for each person for dipping.

PRO TIP: For a lower-carb option, try to find *ssamjang* sauce in your local Asian grocery store as a replacement for gochujang.

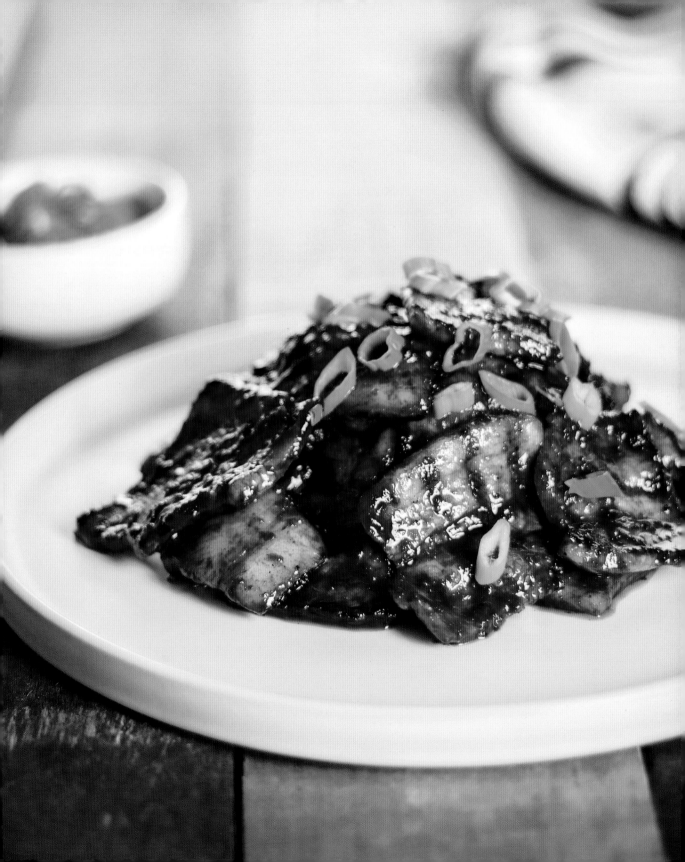

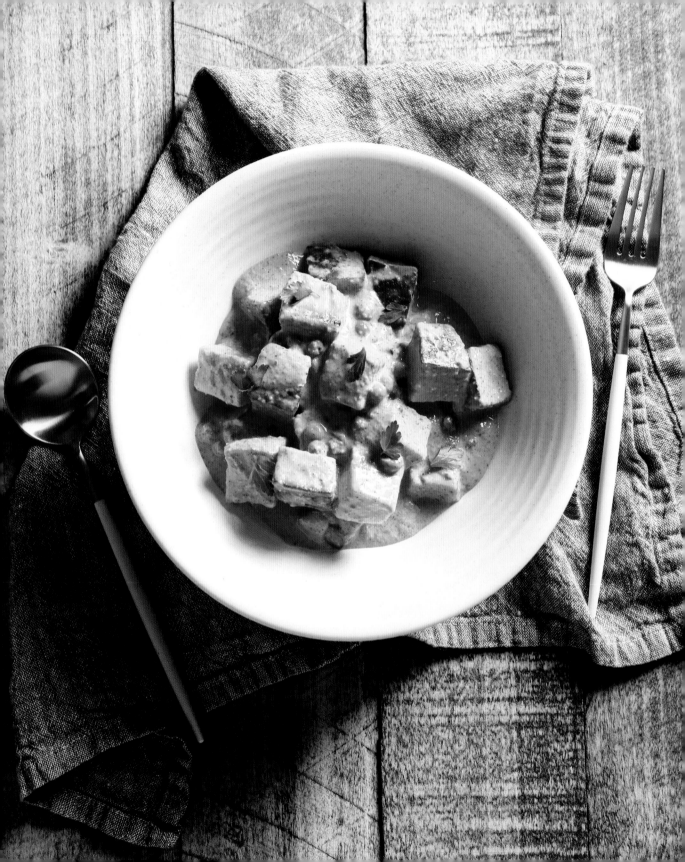

1 lb (455 g) paneer cheese

2 yellow onions, peeled and halved

6 cloves garlic

¼ oz (7 g) fresh ginger (about a 1" [2.5-cm] cube), peeled

¼ cup (58 g) ghee or coconut oil

3 tbsp (18 g) garam masala

2 tsp (5 g) ground turmeric

2 tsp (12 g) kosher salt

1 (14-oz [400-g]) can coconut cream

1 cup (230 g) full-fat Indian or Greek yogurt

3 tbsp (48 g) smooth almond butter

½ cup (65 g) frozen peas

Cilantro leaves, for garnish (optional)

MACROS *per* SERVING

Calories: 852 • Fat: 75.8 g

Carbs: 16.1 g • Net Carbs: 12.9 g

Protein: 26 g

INSTANT POT PANEER KORMA

My trip to India opened my eyes to a new world of food (especially vegetarian food). I could have spent hours in the vast spice markets. In fact, when I left India, I carried back with me several kilograms of spices that I still use today. And while I learned the hard way that large unmarked plastic bags of spices look really suspicious to U.S. Border Patrol, it was all worth it! In Mumbai, I had the most amazing korma curry. Although traditional korma uses ground cashews to thicken the curry, my interpretation uses almond butter instead, as almonds are much lower carb than cashews. But the star here is the paneer, a tasty yet mild nonmelting cheese you can find in most supermarkets today. And if you aren't in the mood for vegetarian, just replace the paneer for cubed chicken or lamb.

Start by cutting the block of paneer into ½-inch (1.3-cm) cubes. Then, in a food processor, combine the onions, garlic and ginger, and blend on high speed until a puree is formed.

In an Instant Pot or other electric pressure cooker on sauté mode, heat the ghee, and once hot, add the onion puree, garam masala, turmeric and salt. Sauté the mixture for 2 minutes to toast the spices. Stir in the coconut cream and cubed paneer. Set the pot to pressure cook on high for 15 minutes. Once done, release the steam, then stir in the yogurt, almond butter and frozen peas. Set the pot back to sauté mode to warm up the peas and yogurt. Once the curry is boiling, it's done. Turn off the heat and serve the korma in a deep bowl. Garnish with fresh cilantro (if using).

DINNERS *to* IMPRESS

WHETHER FOR DATE NIGHT, A HOLIDAY OR ANY occasion, these dishes are designed to pull out your inner chef. And while many of these recipes use techniques common in restaurant kitchens, they are easy enough to make at home. If you want to impress your dinner guests with some truly showstopping Keto dishes, these recipes are the way to do it!

Mike's Signature Crab Cakes (page 70)

Secret-Recipe Whole Roasted Chicken (page 73)

Crispy-Skin Salmon with Brown Butter & Pancetta (page 74)

Filet Mignon with Warm Spinach & Balsamic Reduction (page 77)

Roasted Lamb Rack with Creamy Feta Sauce (page 78)

Cod with Charred Lemon & Braised Leeks (page 81)

Black Pepper Braised Short Ribs (page 82)

Seared Scallops with Pea Puree & Prosciutto Crisps (page 85)

Moroccan Chicken Tagine (page 86)

Korean Beef Bulgogi Ssam (page 89)

Seared Snapper with Wine-Braised Red Cabbage (page 90)

Za'atar-Crusted Chicken & Roasted Carrots (page 93)

Spice-Rubbed Pork Tenderloin with Orange Gastrique (page 94)

5 strips thick-cut bacon

1 lb (455 g) lump USA crabmeat

2 tbsp (28 g) mayonnaise (see Pro Tip)

2 large eggs

1 tbsp (6 g) Old Bay Seasoning

1½ tsp (6 g) Dijon mustard

1 batch Zesty Dill Rémoulade (page 153)

Lemon slices, for garnish (optional)

Fresh dill, for garnish (optional)

MACROS *per* SERVING

Calories: 625 • Fat: 49.8 g

Carbs: 0.6 g • Net Carbs: 0.6 g

Protein: 42 g

MIKE'S SIGNATURE CRAB CAKES

Growing up in Maryland, I'd go crabbing with my dad. We'd spend hours outside over a brown-paper-lined table, carefully plucking every morsel of meat out of dozens of blue crabs (the best crabs in the world!). It's a tradition that is deeply ingrained in who I am. Crab cakes are a part of my culinary journey, and this ketofied version is very special to me. I hope you love them as much as I do.

In a cast-iron skillet over medium heat, cook the bacon for about 3 minutes on each side, or until crispy. Remove the bacon, but leave all the bacon grease. (You can save the bacon for later! We're not using it in the recipe, just the rendered bacon fat in the pan.) Turn off the heat.

In a bowl, combine the crabmeat, mayo, eggs, Old Bay and mustard. Stir gently, but don't overmix, as you do want some of the lumps of crabmeat to remain. Then, using a ⅓-cup (80-ml) measuring cup, form the crab cakes (you should be able to make six or seven cakes) and set them onto a plate (or two plates, as needed).

Reheat your skillet over medium-high heat. Once the bacon fat is hot, carefully drop in your formed crab cakes. DO NOT touch the crab cakes for 2 minutes; they will fall apart if moved too soon. After 2 to 3 minutes, flip them over to the other side. Meanwhile, line a clean plate with paper towels. Once both sides are golden brown, place the crab cakes on the paper towels to drain. Serve them right away, while they're hot and fresh, on a nice plate with a generous spoon swipe of the rémoulade. Garnish with lemon slices and fresh dill (if using).

PRO TIP: For an extra punch of flavor, use the Garlic Aioli (page 141) instead of the store-bought mayo in the recipe.

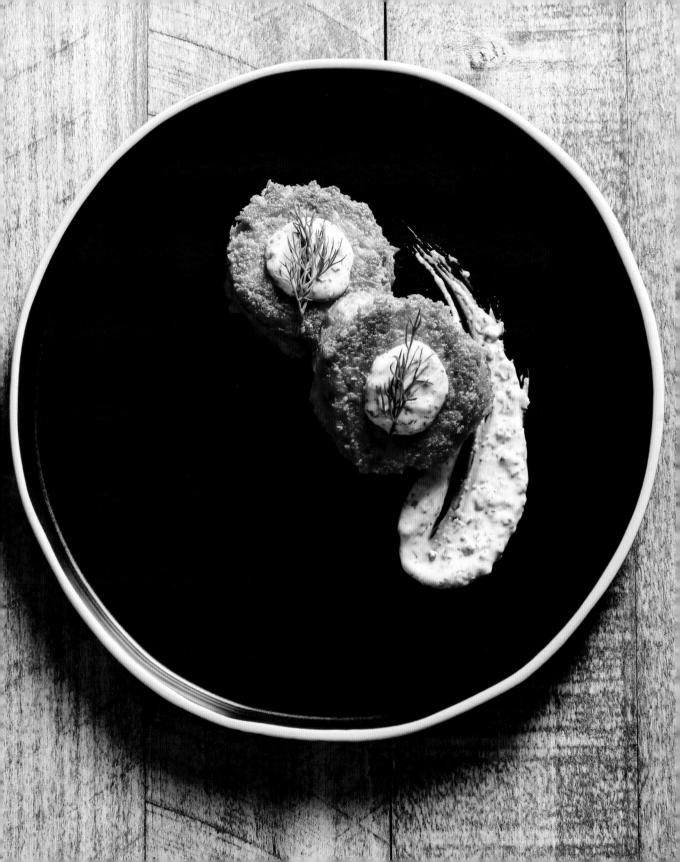

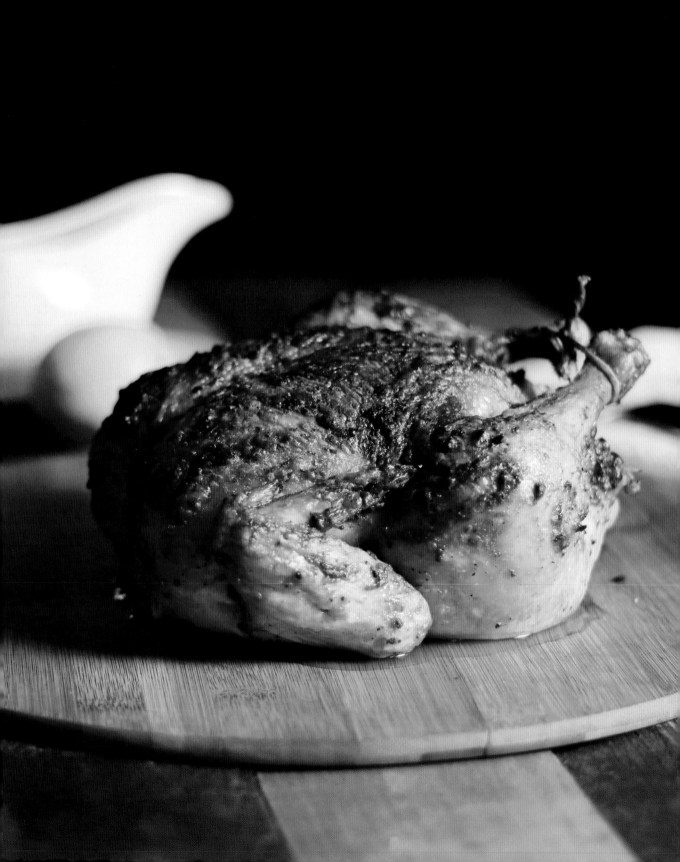

1 (5-lb [2.3-kg]) chicken

½ cup (115 g) mayonnaise

1 tbsp (11 g) Dijon mustard

2 tsp (1 g) herbes de Provence

2 tsp (4 g) garlic powder

1 tsp smoked or sweet paprika

1 tsp dried sage

1 tsp kosher salt

1 tsp freshly ground
black pepper

1 lemon, cut in half

MACROS *per* SERVING

Calories: 691 • Fat: 50.7 g

Carbs: 2.7 g • Net Carbs: 2.5 g

Protein: 56.3 g

SECRET-RECIPE WHOLE ROASTED CHICKEN

There's nothing more impressive than a juicy, flavorful whole roasted chicken. It seems so easy to do, but a perfect chicken is hard to come by. The secret to this one is mayonnaise. The herb-infused mayo rub completely coats this chicken in flavorful goodness and guarantees a juicy chicken every time. This will make a stunning centerpiece at your next holiday dinner.

Try pairing this recipe with the Cheesy Brussels Sprout Gratin (page 102).

Preheat your oven to 400°F (200°C). Remove the chicken from its packaging, remove and discard any giblets and pat the chicken completely dry with paper towels. Let the chicken rest on your counter for 20 minutes to come to room temperature. Line a baking sheet with aluminum foil and place a wire rack on top.

In a small bowl, mix together the mayo, mustard, herbes de Provence, garlic powder, paprika, sage, salt and pepper. Completely coat the chicken with the mayo mixture, ensuring you have evenly covered all sides and between the wings and legs. Be sure to get some of the mayo rub under the skin as well. Place the chicken on the wire rack. Stuff the inside with the lemon halves, and tie the legs together with butcher's twine, or by rolling aluminum foil around the tips of the legs to hold them together. Place in the middle rack of the oven and bake for 80 minutes, or until the thickest part of the meat has an internal temperature of 165°F (73°C).

Remove the chicken from the oven and let it rest for 10 minutes before carving it. I love to serve it whole at the dinner table, as it looks so beautiful at the center of the table.

2 (6-oz [170-g]) skin-on salmon fillets (see Pro Tip)

4 oz (115 g) pancetta or thick-cut bacon, cut into lardons

½ tsp kosher salt

½ cup (112 g or 1 stick) salted butter

1 (1-lb [455-g]) bag fresh haricots verts (a.k.a. French beans)

MACROS *per* SERVING

Calories: 1,046 • Fat: 85.5 g

Carbs: 13.7 g • Net Carbs: 8.2 g

Protein: 52.9 g

CRISPY-SKIN SALMON WITH BROWN BUTTER & PANCETTA

You'll notice this meal doesn't have many ingredients, but using a few restaurant techniques, they turn into something truly special. The perfectly cooked crispy salmon is paired with an incredible brown butter sauce and haricots verts. This elegant dish is full of flavor and healthy fat. You can serve it family style, or plate it up to create a gorgeous dish to impress.

Preheat your oven to 400°F (200°C). Meanwhile, remove the salmon fillets from the fridge and let them rest at room temperature for 30 minutes.

In an oven-safe, nonstick skillet, cook the pancetta over medium-high heat for about 5 minutes, or until crispy. Transfer all of the meat to a plate, but leave the rendered fat in the pan. Place the pan back over high heat.

When it's smoking hot, carefully place the salmon, skin side down, in the pan, and use a weight, such as a small pan, to press down on the fish for exactly 1 minute. Remove the weight, then continue cooking for exactly 2 minutes. While it cooks, salt the meat side of the fish with ¼ teaspoon per fillet. Flip the fillets, so the skin is up, and place the entire pan in the oven. Bake for 4 minutes (5 minutes if you like your salmon more well done). When done, transfer the salmon to a plate to rest.

In a large skillet over high heat, heat the butter, and once melted, cook it for about 2 minutes, or until it turns light brown. Add the haricots verts and sauté for 4 minutes, or just until tender, removing from the heat. Plate the dish by using tongs to place a large bundle of the beans in the center of each of two plates. Drizzle some of the brown butter over the top, add some of the cooked pancetta around the plate and place a fillet of salmon in the center.

PRO TIP: For extra crispy skin, leave your salmon, skin side up, in the fridge, unwrapped, on a plate for 12 to 24 hours before cooking, to dry the skin.

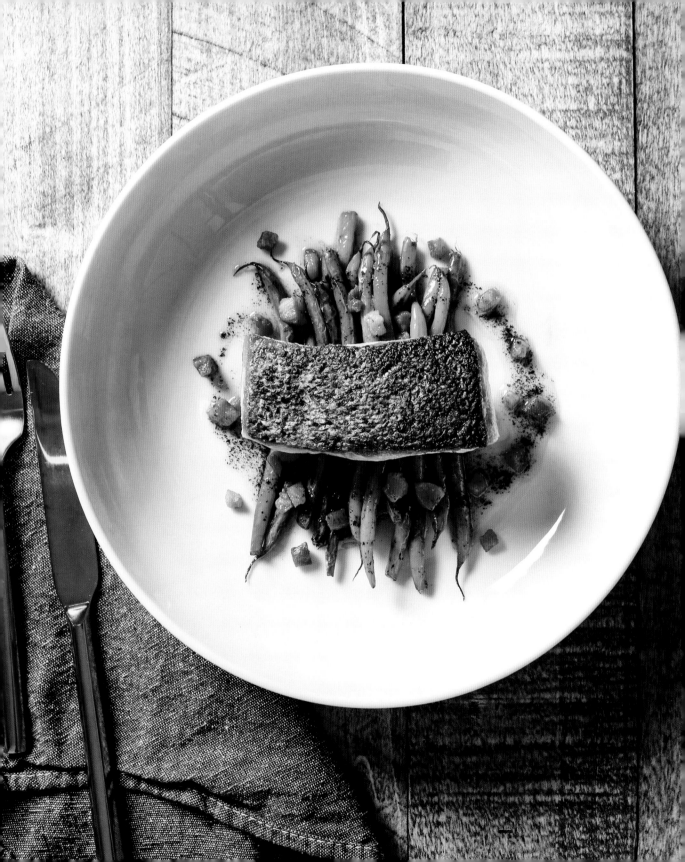

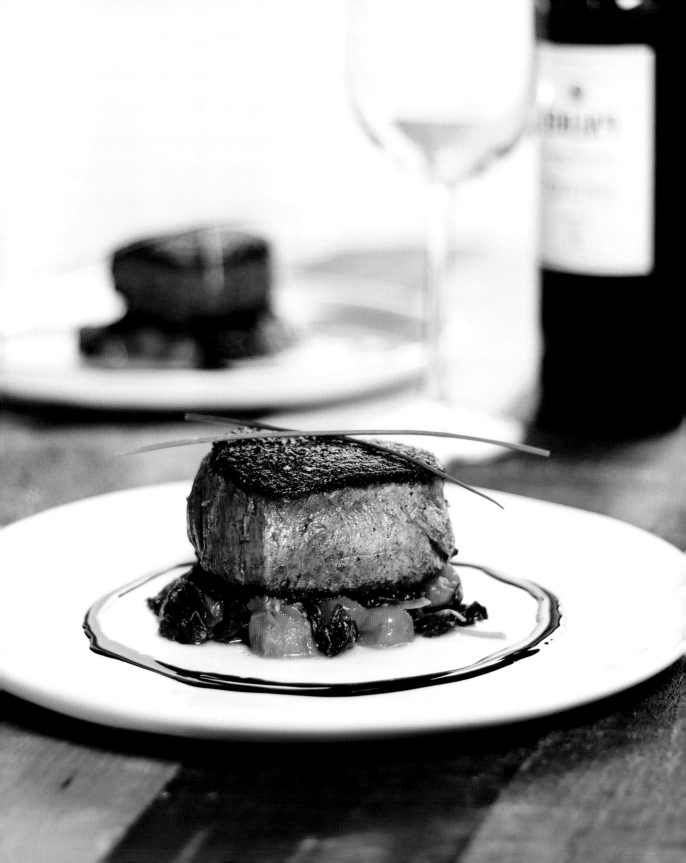

**FILET MIGNON & HOMEMADE
BALSAMIC REDUCTION**

2 (8-oz [225-g]) thick-cut filets mignons,
1½ to 2" (4 to 5 cm) thick

½ cup (120 ml) balsamic vinegar

2 tbsp (30 ml) avocado oil

2 tsp (12 g) kosher salt

1 tsp freshly ground black pepper

¼ cup (57 g or ½ stick) unsalted
butter

3 cloves garlic

2 rosemary sprigs

**WARM SPINACH & TOMATO
SALAD**

2 tbsp (28 g) unsalted butter

2 cloves garlic, finely minced

5 oz (140 g) cherry tomatoes,
cut in half

5 oz (140 g) baby spinach

½ tsp kosher salt

Flake salt, for garnish (I use Maldon
or Falksalt brand)

MACROS *per* SERVING

Calories: 795 • Fat: 59 g

Carbs: 13.1 g • Net Carbs: 11.2 g

Protein: 47.2 g

FILET MIGNON WITH WARM SPINACH & BALSAMIC REDUCTION

This recipe is just a bit fancy, with a whole lotta sexy. Get ready for low-carb elegance.

Try pairing this with The Ultimate Creamy "Risotto" (page 109).

Remove your steak from the fridge and let it rest at room temperature for at least 20 minutes.

Meanwhile, in a saucepan over medium heat, boil the balsamic vinegar for about 10 minutes, stirring occasionally with a rubber spatula. Do not walk away, as it can burn easily. You know it's done when you run the rubber spatula along the bottom, and the sauce momentarily parts and leaves a trail at the bottom of the pan. Remove the pan from the heat and set aside.

In a cast-iron skillet over high heat, heat the avocado oil. Meanwhile, coat each steak with ½ teaspoon of the salt and ¼ teaspoon of the pepper per side. Have the butter, garlic cloves, and rosemary ready, as well as a spoon and an oven mitt. The cooking process happens quickly and it's best to be prepared. Once the pan is smoking hot, cook the steaks on one side for exactly 3 minutes. Flip them over and cook the other side for 2 minutes. Then, immediately add the butter and garlic to the pan, and place a sprig of rosemary on top of each steak. Using the oven mitt, tilt the pan slightly toward you to pool the butter and use the spoon to baste the steaks with butter. After 90 seconds of basting, remove the steaks from the pan and let them rest for 10 minutes.

While the steaks rest, make the spinach salad: In a large, nonstick pan over high heat, heat the butter. Add the minced garlic and fry for 1 minute, then add the cherry tomatoes and sauté for another minute. Add the spinach and salt, and sauté for 30 seconds, stirring constantly, just until the spinach is fully wilted.

Place half of the spinach salad neatly in the center of each of two large dinner plates. Top with a steak, then drizzle the balsamic reduction in a circle around the steak. Garnish the steak with a sprinkle of flake salt.

HERB-CRUSTED RACK OF LAMB

6 cloves garlic

1 tbsp packed (3 g) fresh mint leaves

2 tbsp packed (8 g) fresh parsley leaves

2 tsp (2 g) dried rosemary

1½ tsp (4 g) paprika

1 tbsp (11 g) Dijon mustard

3 tbsp (45 ml) olive oil

1 (1½-lb [680-g]) rack of lamb, frenched

1 tsp kosher salt

½ tsp freshly ground black pepper

CREAMY FETA SAUCE

¼ cup (60 g) mayonnaise

½ cup (115 g) full-fat, plain Greek yogurt

Juice of ½ lemon

4 oz (115 g) feta cheese, in the block (not precrumbled)

MACROS *per* SERVING

Calories: 1,171 • Fat: 77 g

Carbs: 7 g • Net Carbs: 6.7 g

Protein: 106.8 g

ROASTED LAMB RACK WITH CREAMY FETA SAUCE

To me, nothing is more special than a rack of lamb. And though lamb can be intimidating, I designed this recipe to guarantee perfect, juicy results every time. This Mediterranean-inspired dish is perfect for the holidays. The lamb is crusted in a garlicky herb rub and cooked to a perfect medium-rare. The salty and creamy three-ingredient feta sauce is so easy and incredibly tasty and balances the rich flavor of the lamb. If you can't find the lamb rack already "frenched," just ask the butcher to do it for you.

Try pairing this with the Lemony Charred Broccolini (page 106).

Prepare the lamb: Preheat your oven to 475°F (240°C) and place a wire rack on a baking sheet. In a food processor, combine the garlic, mint, parsley, rosemary, paprika, mustard and olive oil. Blend on high speed until a paste forms. Set the herb paste aside in a bowl. Rinse the food processor clean, as you will need it for the yogurt sauce.

Remove the lamb rack from the fridge and slice off and discard any excess fat on top. A thin layer is okay, as that keeps the lamb moist and juicy, but remove as much as you can without damaging the meat. Dust each side of the lamb with ½ teaspoon of salt and ¼ teaspoon of pepper. Then, evenly spread the herb paste all over the meat using the back of a spoon. Place the lamb on the prepared baking sheet and bake for 30 to 35 minutes, or until the internal temperature is 125°F (51°C) (see Pro Tip).

While the lamb cooks, make the feta sauce: In the clean food processor, combine the mayo, yogurt, lemon juice and feta cheese. Pulse until the sauce is combined. I like to leave some of the feta visibly chunky in the sauce, but you can blend on high speed until smooth, if desired.

Once the lamb is cooked, remove it from the oven and let it rest for 10 minutes before carving it into double-cut chops (slice between every other bone). Serve with a bed of sauce on a beautiful plate.

PRO TIP: Each lamb rack will be a slightly different size, so cooking times are estimated here. To ensure a perfectly cooked lamb rack, use a meat thermometer.

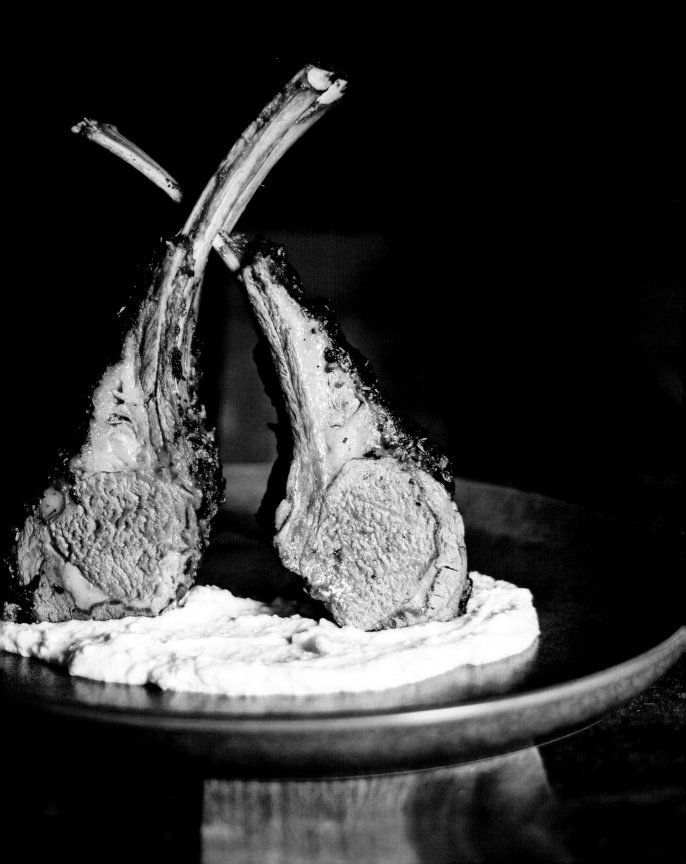

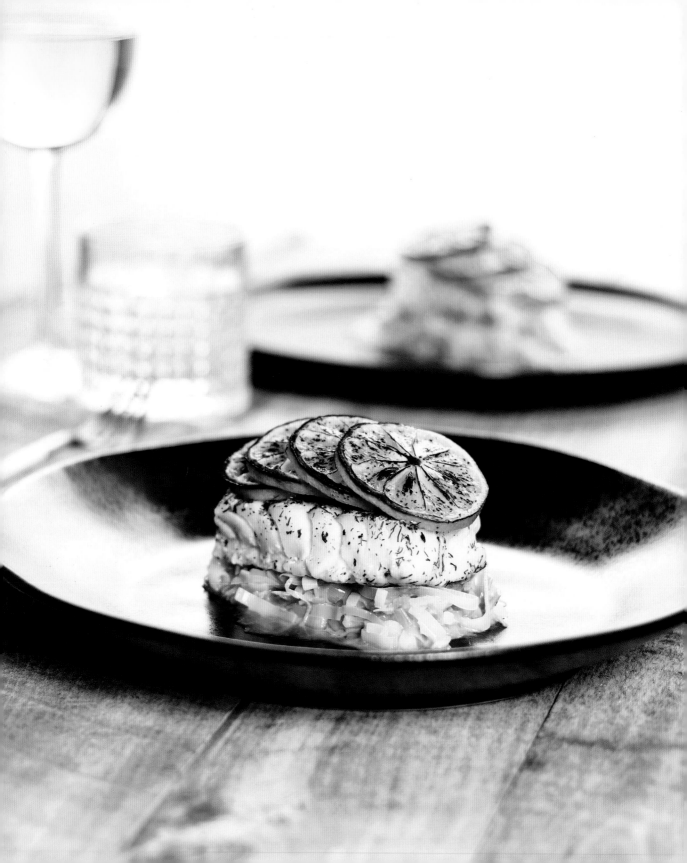

BRAISED LEEKS

2 lb (905 g) leeks

6 tbsp (84 g or ¾ stick) unsalted butter

4 cloves garlic, minced

½ tsp kosher salt

1 cup (240 ml) dry white wine

COD WITH CHARRED LEMON

2 (8-oz [225-g]) cod fillets

2 lemons

1 tbsp (15 ml) olive oil

1 tsp kosher salt

½ tsp freshly ground black pepper

½ tsp smoked or sweet paprika

½ tsp dried dill

½ tsp dried basil

MACROS *per* SERVING

Calories: 780 • Fat: 43.5 g

Carbs: 19.6 g • Net Carbs: 17.4 g

Protein: 54.6 g

COD WITH CHARRED LEMON & BRAISED LEEKS

Cod is such a mild fish, so I wanted to pair it with some big fat Greek flavors. The braised leeks are slow cooked in butter, garlic and white wine, so you just know those are going to be tasty. The charred lemon is not only beautiful, it keeps the fish incredibly juicy and flavorful.

Preheat your oven to 425°F (220°C). Prepare the oven so one oven rack is in the middle and the other rack is on the very top. Line a small rimmed baking sheet or roasting pan with aluminum foil for easy cleanup.

Prepare the leeks: Slice off all the dark green stems from the leeks, then slice off the root tips, leaving only the 5 inches (12.5 cm) of light green round stems. Discard just the first outer layer from the stems and rinse the leeks of any dirt. Slice them into ⅛-inch (3-mm) rings, then set them aside. In a saucepan (with a lid) over high heat, heat the butter and garlic. Sauté the garlic for 1 minute, then add the leeks and salt. Sauté for another minute, then add the wine. Stir well, then bring the mixture to a boil, place the lid on the pot, turn the heat down to medium-low and simmer for 35 minutes, stirring occasionally.

Prepare the cod: When the leeks have cooked for about 15 minutes, remove the fish from the fridge and leave it on your countertop for about 10 minutes to come to room temperature. Thinly slice the lemons into rings. Add the olive oil to the prepared baking sheet and roll the fish in the olive oil. Evenly coat all sides of the fish with the salt, pepper, paprika, dill and basil. Then, layer the lemon slices over the top of the fish, almost like scales, covering the entire fillet. Place the pan on the middle baking rack and bake for 5 minutes (7 minutes if your fillets are thick). As soon as the time is up, switch your oven to broil and move the pan of fish to the top rack. Set a timer for 5 minutes, and don't walk away. Let the broiler char the lemons. It may start to smoke, but watch carefully as you don't want a fire. After 5 minutes, remove the fish from the oven.

To plate, place a large spoonful of leeks on the center of each of two plates, then carefully place a fillet on top.

1½ tsp (9 g) kosher salt

2 tbsp (13 g) freshly ground black pepper (see Pro Tip)

1 tbsp (9 g) garlic powder

1½ tsp (4 g) smoked paprika (or chipotle powder, if you want them spicy!)

2½ lb (1.1 kg) bone-in short ribs ("English Cut"; 3 to 4" [7.5 to 10 cm] long)

2 tbsp (30 ml) avocado oil

1 cup (240 ml) dry red wine

½ cup (120 ml) beef stock

1 tbsp (15 ml) balsamic vinegar

2 rosemary sprigs

MACROS *per* SERVING

Calories: 1,004 • Fat: 76.9 g

Carbs: 4.8 g • Net Carbs: 4.8 g

Protein: 55.5 g

BLACK PEPPER BRAISED SHORT RIBS

Thanks to the Instant Pot, these tender short ribs are a showstopper. The rich flavors from the red wine and black pepper will blow your dinner guests away. This spectacular dish is perfect for a date or that special holiday meal with family. This recipe proves that you can get fancy in the kitchen and make it look easy!

This goes perfectly with The Perfect Mashed "Faux-tatoes" (page 101).

In a small bowl, mix together the salt, pepper, garlic powder and smoked paprika. Place the short ribs on a large plate and completely coat all sides of the ribs with the spice rub by pressing the rub into the meat. Make sure you use nearly all of the spice mixture, as you really want a good crust on the ribs.

Turn your Instant Pot or electric pressure cooker to sauté mode and add the avocado oil. Once it's smoking hot, brown the ribs, meat side down, for 3 to 4 minutes, to get a dark brown color on the crust. You do not need to sear the "bone" side. If your ribs don't all fit, brown them in batches. Once the meat is browned, add the red wine, beef stock, balsamic vinegar and rosemary sprigs to the pot. Set the pot to high pressure, close the lid and cook for 45 minutes.

After 45 minutes, turn off the pot. For extra tender meat, do not release the pressure. Let it slowly cool and depressurize on its own. If you need a shortcut, you can release the pressure immediately, but the ribs will not be as tender. Once the pressure is released, open the lid. Carefully remove the ribs with tongs and set them aside on a plate. Loosely cover the plate with aluminum foil to keep them warm.

To make the gravy, pour the remaining broth through a fine-mesh strainer directly into a large skillet. Place the skillet over high heat and bring the broth to a boil. Simmer for 8 to 10 minutes, stirring constantly. The broth will reduce and thicken. Place the ribs on a beautiful plate and pour the gravy over the top to serve.

PRO TIP: For maximum flavor, crack your own black pepper in a mortar and pestle. The pepper is the star of this dish, so you want as much flavor as possible.

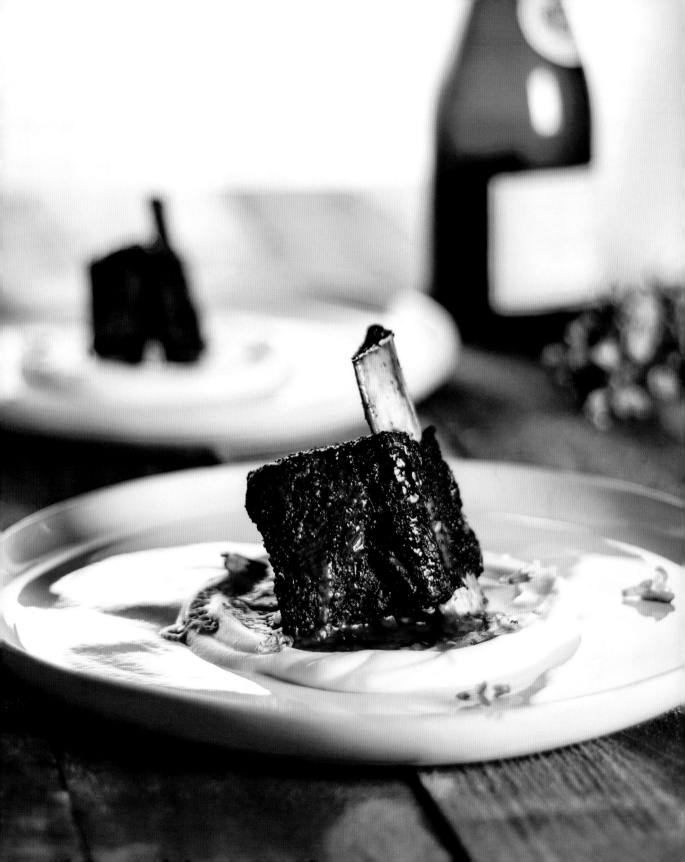

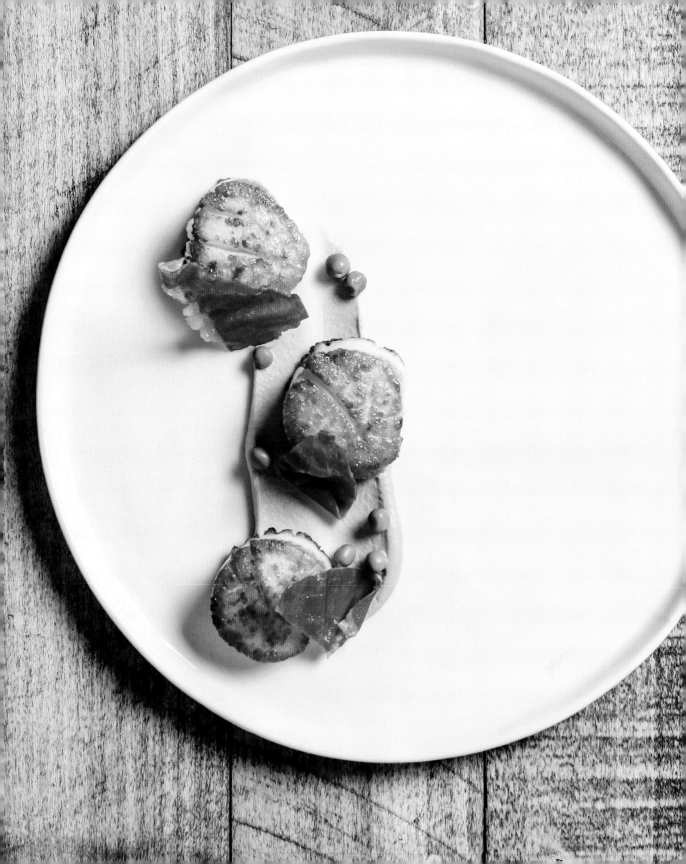

SEARED SCALLOPS

12 oz (340 g) fresh sea scallops (large size)

2 tbsp (30 ml) avocado oil

½ tsp kosher salt

PEA PUREE & PROSCIUTTO CRISPS

4 cups (946 ml) water

1 tbsp (18 g) plus ⅛ tsp kosher salt, divided

8 oz (225 g) fresh English peas

2 tbsp (28 g) unsalted butter

½ cup (120 ml) heavy whipping cream

2 oz (55 g) prosciutto

MACROS *per* SERVING

Calories: 713 • Fat: 52.5 g

Carbs: 17.1 g • Net Carbs: 13.1 g

Protein: 43.4 g

PRO TIP: For an extra smooth and creamy pea puree, use a high-powered blender, such as a Vitamix. If you don't have one, after blending, press your puree through a wire-mesh sieve instead.

SEARED SCALLOPS WITH PEA PUREE & PROSCIUTTO CRISPS

Another date night favorite in my house, this recipe walks you through how to sear the perfect sea scallops, as well as how to make a beautifully smooth pea puree. The prosciutto chips are a fun bonus recipe you can use to make a yummy snack anytime. This sexy dish will top any high-end restaurant meal you can get and will definitely impress your date.

Try pairing this with the Jicama & Orange Slaw (page 113).

Preheat your oven to 350°F (180°C). Remove the scallops from the fridge. Remove the small adductor muscle on the side of the scallops, if present, and dry them with a paper towel. Let them sit at room temperature for 20 to 30 minutes.

Meanwhile, make the pea puree: In a small saucepan, bring the water and the tablespoon (18 g) of salt to a boil. Once the water is rapidly boiling, add the peas. Boil them for 10 minutes, then drain. Remove from the pan and set aside 2 tablespoons (10 g) of the peas, to use later as garnish, and then place the rest of the peas in a blender along with the butter, cream and remaining ⅛ teaspoon of salt. Blend on high speed for 2 to 3 minutes, scraping the sides of the blender as needed, until the puree is velvety smooth. Set aside.

To make the prosciutto chips, simply lay slices of prosciutto on a cookie sheet and bake them at 350°F (180°C) for 15 minutes. Let them cool completely and then break them into shards.

Cook the scallops: In a large, nonstick skillet, heat the avocado oil over high heat. Salt the scallops on both sides with the ½ teaspoon of salt. Once the pan is smoking hot (you really want the pan very hot), gently add the scallops. Sear, without touching them, for 90 seconds. Flip them over and sear on the other side for another 90 seconds. Remove them from the pan and place them on a plate to rest.

To plate the dish, add the pea puree to the plate in a spoon swipe. Add the scallops in a line, then garnish with the prosciutto crisps and reserved whole peas.

2 white onions

1 zucchini (about 10 oz [280 g])

1 yellow summer squash (about 8 oz [225 g])

8 cloves garlic

1½ tbsp (11 g) sweet or smoked paprika

1½ tsp (4 g) ground cinnamon

½ tsp ground ginger

¼ tsp cayenne pepper or red pepper flakes (optional)

2 lb (905 g) bone-in, skin-on chicken legs

2 tsp (12 g) kosher salt, divided

3 tbsp (45 ml) avocado oil, divided

1 cup (240 ml) low-sodium chicken stock

½ cup (50 g) pitted green olives

1 lemon, cut in half (see Pro Tip)

Chopped fresh parsley, for garnish (optional)

MACROS *per* SERVING

Calories: 432 • Fat: 27.8 g

Carbs: 10.6 g • Net Carbs: 8.8 g

Protein: 34.5 g

MOROCCAN CHICKEN TAGINE

Many years ago, I learned this dish from the chef at a Moroccan restaurant I worked at in my twenties. I found the flavors to be bright and vibrant, and I was really inspired by this cuisine. And while this recipe has a lot of ingredients, it's surprisingly easy to make. The mix of spices, especially the use of cinnamon, not commonly used in savory cooking, makes this dish really quite special. Of course, you don't need a tagine (the cone-shaped clay pot) to cook this dish, but it sure is pretty!

Preheat your oven to 400°F (200°C). Meanwhile, slice the onions into thin half-rounds, chop the zucchini and squash into bite-size quarter-rounds, rough chop the garlic, then set all the veggies aside. In a small bowl, combine the paprika, cinnamon, ginger and cayenne (if using), to make a spice blend. Coat all sides of the chicken legs with 1½ teaspoons (9 g) of the salt.

In a large Dutch oven or tagine over high heat, heat 2 tablespoons (30 ml) of the avocado oil. Once hot, sear the chicken for 2 minutes on each side to get a nice crust. Remove the chicken to a plate. Add another tablespoon (15 ml) of oil and the onions to the pot, and sauté for about 4 minutes, or until the onions are slightly translucent. Add the chopped garlic and spice blend, and sauté for 1 minute, then add the chicken stock and remaining ½ teaspoon of salt. Stir the bottom of the pan to remove all the fond, then add the zucchini, squash and olives. Squeeze the lemon juice into the pot, and add the lemon halves as well. Stir well and then nestle the chicken on top. Cover the pot and bake for 30 minutes. Garnish with chopped parsley (if using) and serve family style.

PRO TIP: Try replacing the lemon with ⅓ cup (83 g) of chopped preserved lemon, rind included, for an authentic Moroccan touch.

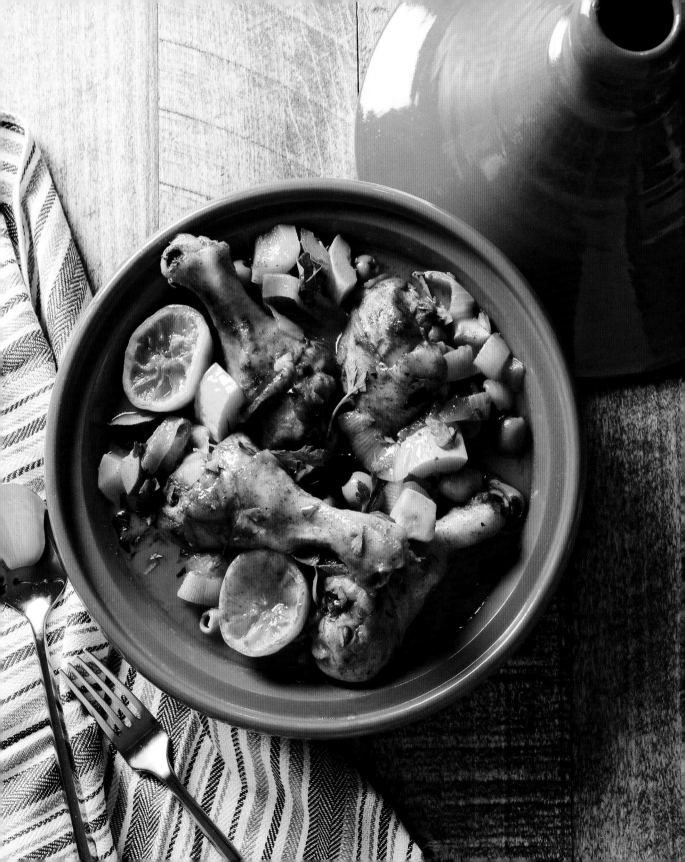

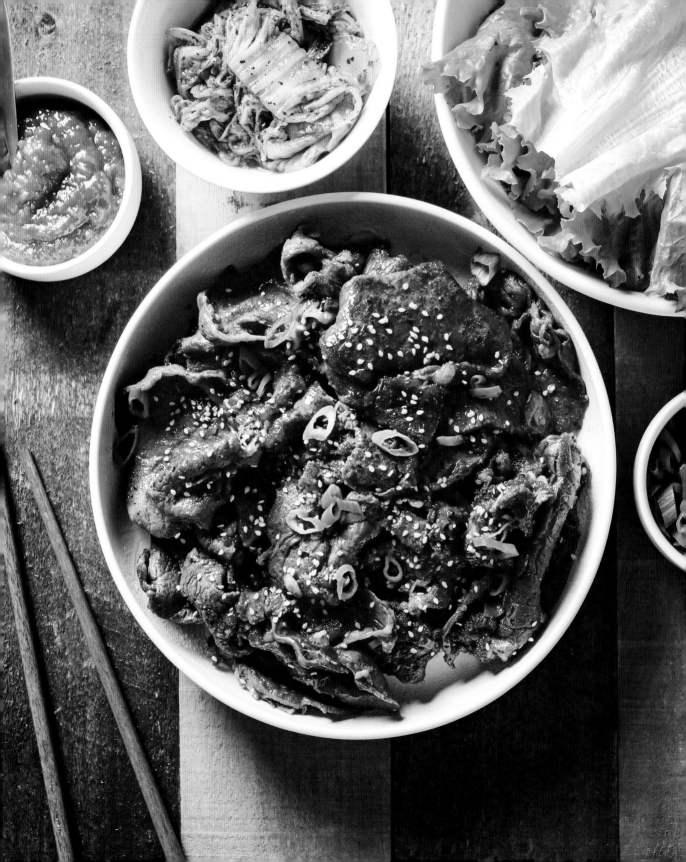

6 cloves garlic

⅓ oz (10 g) peeled fresh ginger

8 scallions

½ cup (120 ml) low-sodium soy sauce

5 tbsp (75 ml) sesame oil

¼ cup (48 g) allulose sweetener

1 tsp freshly ground black pepper

2 lb (905 g) ribeye steak, very thinly shaved (see Pro Tip)

1 tsp sesame seeds

1 head green leaf lettuce, separated into leaves

Gochujang or ssamjang sauce, for serving (optional)

MACROS *per* SERVING

Calories: 631 ● Fat: 37.9 g

Carbs: 5.7 g ● Net Carbs: 5.1 g

Protein: 67.7 g

KOREAN BEEF BULGOGI SSAM

Korean BBQ is among my favorite foods in the world, and this recipe brings it right to your kitchen. Ssam, also known as Korean lettuce wraps, are the perfect Keto treat for the whole family. The shaved steak is marinated in a simple salty and sweet sauce, and then served with lettuce leaves and tasty sides. You can serve this with cauliflower rice, too. It's a really nice way to introduce your friends and family to a fun, hands-on Korean dinner.

Using a small hand grater or microplane, grate the garlic to a paste. Then, grate 1 packed teaspoon (about 4 g) of fresh ginger. Very thinly slice the scallions into rings, setting aside a few tablespoons (about 6 g) of the dark green tops for garnish. In a large bowl, combine the garlic, ginger and scallions along with the soy sauce, sesame oil, allulose and black pepper. Mix well, then add the shaved steak. Use tongs to toss the steak in the marinade. Cover the bowl with plastic wrap and let it marinate for at least 30 minutes (the longer you marinate, the better).

Using a large wok or skillet over high heat, spread an even layer of the steak mixture on the cooking surface. Let it cook for 3 minutes, and then flip and cook for 2 to 3 more minutes, or until the steak is just cooked. Do not stir the steak while it's cooking, as we want to sear the steak and build up color. Once it's done, place the steak on a large platter and garnish with the reserved scallions and sesame seeds. Serve with lettuce leaves to make lettuce wraps, and make sure to have gochujang or *ssamjang* sauce (if using) to spread on the lettuce wraps for traditional Korean-style ssam.

PRO TIP: You can always find shaved ribeye for bulgogi at an Asian market. However, most supermarkets have shaved steak for cheesesteaks that also works here.

BRAISED CABBAGE

½ small head red cabbage (about 1 lb [455 g]; save the other half for another recipe, such as Jicama & Orange Slaw [page 113])

¼ cup (57 g or ½ stick) unsalted butter

½ cup (120 ml) dry red wine

¼ cup (60 ml) balsamic vinegar

¼ tsp kosher salt

SEARED SNAPPER

2 (6-oz [170-g]) skin-on red snapper fillets, scaled and deboned

½ tsp kosher salt, divided

2 tbsp (30 ml) avocado oil

¼ tsp freshly ground black pepper

1 batch Garlic Aioli (page 141)

Microgreens, fresh chervil or fennel fronds, for garnish (optional)

MACROS *per* SERVING

Calories: 729 • Fat: 48.6 g

Carbs: 16.6 g • Net Carbs: 14.7 g

Protein: 44.5 g

SEARED SNAPPER WITH WINE-BRAISED RED CABBAGE

This elegant meal is surprisingly easy. The simply seared snapper goes incredibly well with the wine-braised cabbage, which becomes naturally sweet as the wine and balsamic vinegar reduce. And though it's not necessary, trust me, you want to make the Garlic Aioli (page 141) for this recipe. It takes this dish to new heights.

Prepare the cabbage: Remove the thick stem and then shave the cabbage into thin strips (as you would for coleslaw). In a large saucepan over medium heat, melt the butter. Add the cabbage and stir to coat with the butter. Sauté the cabbage for about 10 minutes, then add the wine, balsamic vinegar and kosher salt. Place a lid on the pot and let it braise for at least 20 minutes, or until the cabbage has absorbed all the liquid and is tender.

Once the cabbage is done, prepare the snapper: Heat a nonstick skillet over high heat. Pat the snapper fillets dry with a paper towel, then spread ¼ teaspoon of the salt on the skin side of the fish. Have ready a smaller, heavy-bottomed skillet or grill press to use to weigh down the fish. Once the nonstick skillet is smoking hot, add the avocado oil, then add the fish, skin side down, and immediately use the smaller pan to press the fish flat on the pan. Cook for exactly 2 minutes. Remove the top pan and sprinkle the flesh side with the remaining ¼ teaspoon of salt and the pepper. Then, flip it over and cook the fish for 2 more minutes. Place it on a plate to rest.

Plate this dish by doing a swipe of aioli, adding about 1 cup (150 g) of cabbage on top of the sauce and a fillet on top. Garnish with microgreens, some fresh chervil or fennel fronds (if using).

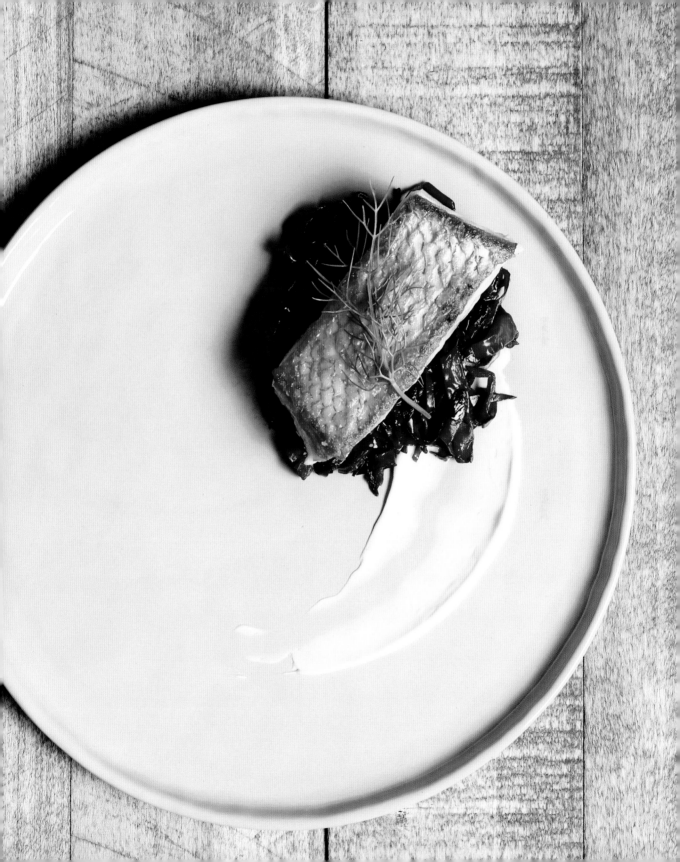

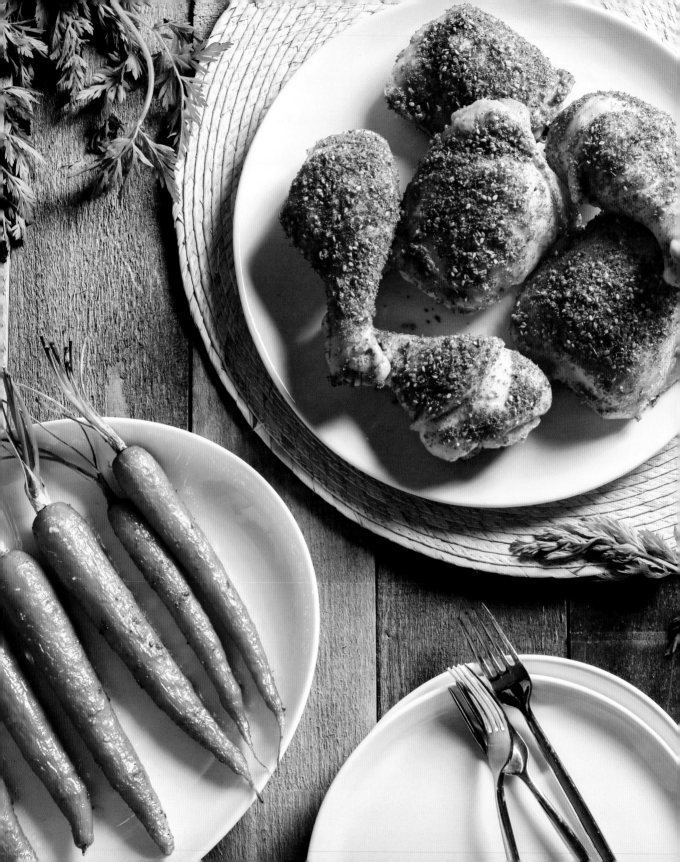

1½ lb (680 g) bone-in, skin-on chicken thighs

1½ lb (680 g) bone-in, skin-on chicken legs

1 lb (455 g) whole carrots with tops (rainbow carrots, if available)

2 tbsp (30 ml) olive oil

2 tsp (12 g) kosher salt, divided

3 tbsp (23 g) za'atar seasoning

1 batch Easy Tahini Yogurt Sauce (page 149; optional)

MACROS *per* SERVING

Calories: 666 • Fat: 39.2 g

Carbs: 12.5 g • Net Carbs: 8.1 g

Protein: 64.3 g

ZA'ATAR-CRUSTED CHICKEN & ROASTED CARROTS

Za'atar is a popular Middle Eastern spice blend that I first came across on a trip to Israel. It's packed with various herbs, sesame seeds and sumac, and it brings a truly special herbal flavor that I fell in love with. This sheet pan meal couldn't be easier and will introduce your dinner guests to some exciting new flavors.

Preheat your oven to 425°F (220°C). Line a baking sheet with aluminum foil. Remove the chicken from your fridge and pat it dry with paper towels. Remove the carrot tops, leaving 1 to 2 inches (2.5 to 5 cm) of the stems attached, and place them on the prepared baking sheet. Pour the olive oil and ½ teaspoon of the salt on top of the carrots, and toss them well. Then, spread them out on the baking sheet, leaving spaces for the chicken pieces.

Place the chicken on the baking sheet and roll them in the residual olive oil on the pan. Then, evenly coat both sides of the chicken with the remaining 1½ teaspoons (9 g) of salt. Leave the chicken skin side up and evenly coat the top and sides of the chicken with the za'atar seasoning. Bake for 35 minutes. Then, turn your oven to broil and toast the top of the chicken and carrots for 3 to 5 minutes. Keep an eye on the oven, as the top can easily burn. Remove from the oven to rest. Serve the carrots and chicken on large platters, with the tahini yogurt sauce, if desired, for a beautiful family-style meal.

PRO TIP: Don't throw away those carrot tops—they're edible! Use them instead of basil to make a tasty carrot-top pesto.

SERVES 2

SPICE-RUBBED PORK TENDERLOIN

1 lb (455 g) pork tenderloin

1 tsp smoked paprika (for a spicy version, use chipotle powder)

2 tsp (5 g) sweet paprika

½ tsp ground ginger

½ tsp garlic powder

1 tsp kosher salt

1 tsp freshly ground black pepper

3 tbsp (45 ml) avocado oil

ORANGE GASTRIQUE

½ cup (120 ml) fresh orange juice

3 tbsp (45 ml) cider vinegar (I prefer Bragg organic)

¼ cup (48 g) allulose sweetener

1 rosemary sprig

1½ tsp (10 g) sugar-free orange marmalade

MACROS *per* SERVING

Calories: 602 • Fat: 35.9 g

Carbs: 7.4 g • Net Carbs: 7.1 g

Protein: 59.7 g

SPICE-RUBBED PORK TENDERLOIN WITH ORANGE GASTRIQUE

This dish is an homage to my grandmother, Nana Shirley, who made pork chops with sweet-and-sour sauce. This version uses oranges to bring beautiful fruity flavors and natural sweetness to the sauce, but without the added sugar. The fresh rosemary brings a floral note, while the spice rub on the pork supplies heat and nutty flavors. This is a modern take on a classic, and you'll be licking the plate clean.

Try pairing this with the Jicama & Orange Slaw (page 113).

Prepare the pork: Preheat your oven to 350°F (180°C). Remove the pork tenderloin from the fridge and pat it dry with a paper towel. Set it aside. In a small bowl, combine the smoked paprika, sweet paprika, ginger, garlic powder, salt and pepper. Completely coat the tenderloin with the spice mixture. You want to press the spices into the meat on all sides.

In a large, cast-iron skillet over high heat, heat the avocado oil. Once it's smoking hot, sear the pork by cooking each side, rotating 90 degrees every 30 seconds. After you've seared all four sides of the pork, place the entire skillet in the oven and bake for about 15 minutes, or until the internal temperature at the center is 130°F (54°C) (see Pro Tip). Remove the pork from the pan and let it rest on a cutting board for 10 minutes before carving into slices.

Prepare the gastrique: In a small saucepan, combine the orange juice and vinegar. Cook over medium-high heat until the mixture reduces to about half of its original volume. Add the allulose and rosemary sprig, and bring the sauce to a boil. Cook for another minute; the sauce will begin to thicken. Remove the pot from the heat, remove the rosemary sprig and add the marmalade. As it cools, the sauce will become thick and velvety. Once the sauce is ready, plate the dish by drizzling the sauce onto the plate and fanning out the slices of pork on top.

PRO TIP: To guarantee a perfectly juicy pork tenderloin, use a meat thermometer. It's a perfect medium-rare at 130°F (54°C).

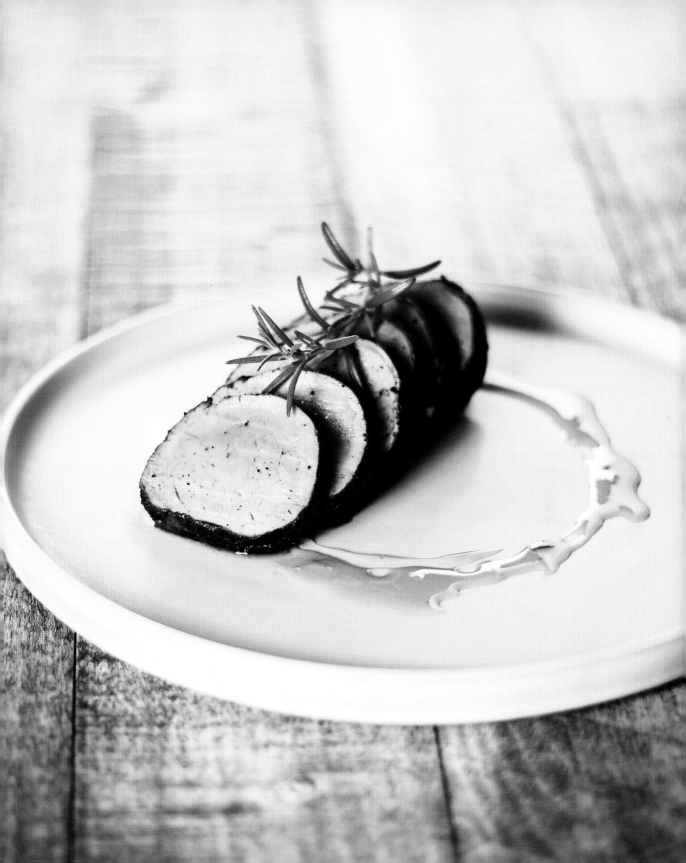

VEGGIES & SIDES

IF YOU'RE ANYTHING LIKE ME, THEN YOU KNOW THAT side dishes are the best part of the meal. And these sides are not to be forgotten. These recipes make veggies the star of the show and pair perfectly with so many of the entrées in this book. Pick a dinner recipe and pair it with one or two of these sides for the perfect party spread.

Grilled Asparagus with Feta & Pistachio (page 98)

The Perfect Mashed "Faux-tatoes" (page 101)

Cheesy Brussels Sprout Gratin (page 102)

Herb-Roasted Kabocha Squash (page 105)

Lemony Charred Broccolini (page 106)

The Ultimate Creamy "Risotto" (page 109)

Button Mushroom Flambé (page 110)

Jicama & Orange Slaw (page 113)

1 lb (455 g) asparagus

2 tbsp (30 ml) olive oil

½ tsp kosher salt

2 tbsp (16 g) pistachios

1 oz (28 g) feta cheese, in the block (not precrumbled)

½ lemon

MACROS *per* SERVING

Calories: 14 • Fat: 6.1 g

Carbs: 8.3 g • Net Carbs: 4.4 g

Protein: 6.1 g

GRILLED ASPARAGUS WITH FETA & PISTACHIO

Sometimes simple is better. And something as simple as asparagus can be truly memorable just by adding a couple key ingredients. These Mediterranean flavors pair perfectly with the smoky grilled asparagus. The feta brings a creaminess and saltiness, while the pistachio brings texture to the dish.

Try this at your next barbecue or paired with Mike's Signature Crab Cakes (page 70).

Heat your grill or cast-iron grill pan to high heat. While it's warming up, slice off the 1 inch (2.5 cm) of fibrous ends of the asparagus. Toss the asparagus in the olive oil and salt. Then, take a ziplock bag and add the pistachios. Use a rolling pin or skillet to smash the pistachios into crumbs. In a small bowl, crumble the feta cheese by hand.

Once the grill is smoking hot, add the asparagus and cook for about 4 minutes, flipping halfway through. Transfer the asparagus to a large plate. Squeeze a bit of lemon juice over the top, sprinkle with crumbled feta and top with the crushed pistachios.

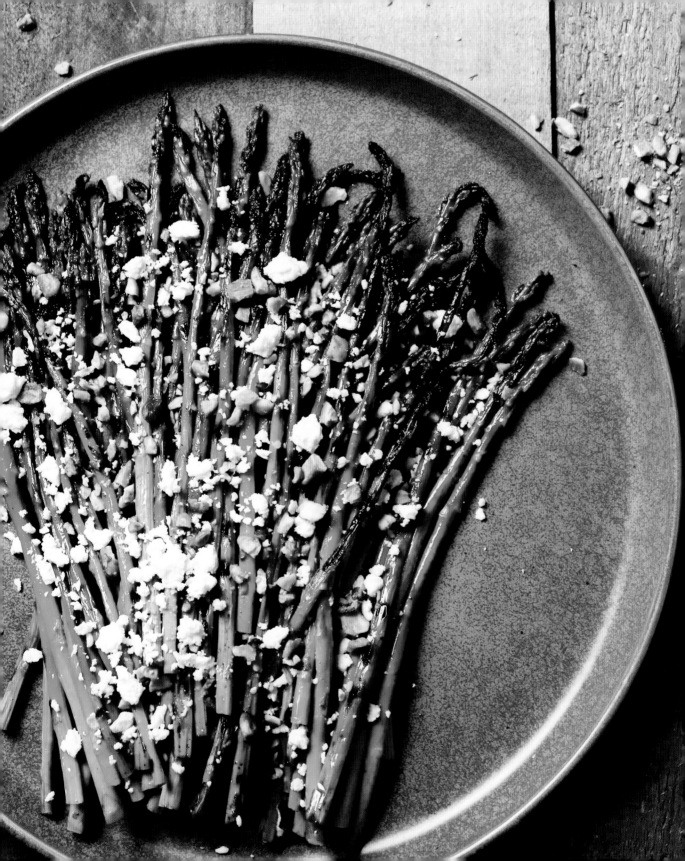

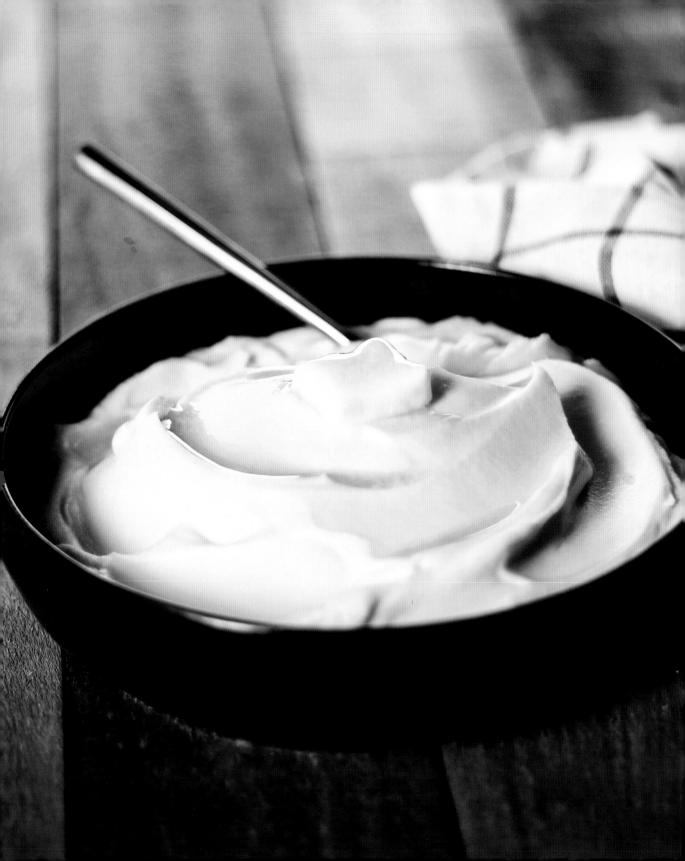

2 lb (905 g) celery root (a.k.a. celeriac)

2 tbsp (37 g) plus 1 tsp kosher salt, divided

¾ cup (175 ml) heavy whipping cream

¼ cup (57 g or ½ stick) unsalted butter, plus an extra slice for garnish

¼ tsp ground white pepper

1 clove garlic, finely minced

MACROS *per* SERVING

Calories: 168 • Fat: 15.3 g

Carbs: 7.4 g • Net Carbs: 6.1 g

Protein: 1.6 g

THE PERFECT MASHED "FAUX-TATOES"

What I love about the Keto diet is that I've never felt deprived. These creamy, buttery "faux-tatoes" leave nothing to be desired. This new version of a classic tastes just like the real thing, but without all the carbs. Make this for your friends and family; just don't tell them it's celery root. Trust me, they'll never know!

I love to pair these with Black Pepper Braised Short Ribs (page 82).

In a large saucepan, bring 12 cups (2.8 L) of water to a boil over high heat. While the water is heating, peel the celery root by running a knife around the outside. Remove all of the brown skin and any imperfections, then roughly cut the celery root into 1-inch (2.5-cm) cubes. Using a kitchen scale, check that you have 1½ pounds (680 g) of cleaned, peeled celery root remaining.

Once the water is boiling, add 2 tablespoons (37 g) of kosher salt to the water, plus the cut celery root. Cover the pot and lower the heat to medium-high. Cook the celery root for 15 minutes—you want it very soft (fork-tender). Once the celery root is cooked, drain it in a colander. Do not rinse.

In a large blender, combine the cream, butter, remaining teaspoon of salt, white pepper, minced garlic and cooked celery root. Pulse the blender several times until no more large lumps are visible, stirring with a rubber spatula as needed. Then, blend on high speed for a full minute. When done, it will be velvety smooth. If your blender is small, you may need to do this in two batches. If your blender is having trouble mixing, try adding an extra tablespoon or two (15 to 30 ml) of cream to thin out the mixture. Serve in a bowl with an extra slice of butter to melt over the top.

6 strips bacon (5 oz [140 g])

2 (10-oz [280-g]) bags shaved Brussels sprouts

4 cloves garlic, minced

1 tsp kosher salt

1 tsp freshly ground black pepper

4 scallions, thinly sliced

2 cups (475 ml) heavy whipping cream

1½ cups (150 g) shredded Italian blend cheese, divided

½ cup (40 g) shredded Parmesan cheese

MACROS *per* SERVING

Calories: 359 • Fat: 30.9 g

Carbs: 9.6 g • Net Carbs: 6.9 g

Protein: 11.9 g

CHEESY BRUSSELS SPROUT GRATIN

These creamed Brussels sprouts are the ultimate in comfort food. If you need to trick your family into eating more veggies, this is the way to do it. Think of this as healthy mac and cheese! The creamy sauce is garlicky and delicious, and the bacon gives this dish a sweet and smoky flavor that takes this over the top. This low-carb side dish goes perfectly with chicken, steak or salmon. And you can also make it a day or two ahead, and just reheat it in the oven.

Try pairing this with the Secret-Recipe Whole Roasted Chicken (page 73).

Preheat your oven to broil. In a large, cast-iron skillet, fry the bacon for about 5 minutes, or until crispy. Remove the bacon and set it aside, but leave the bacon fat in the pan. Lower the heat to medium and add the shaved Brussels sprouts, garlic, salt and pepper. Sauté the Brussels for 2 minutes. Add the sliced scallions, cream and 1 cup (100 g) of the shredded Italian blend cheese. Stir well to combine, then let everything simmer for 6 minutes, stirring every minute. Top the skillet with the remaining ½ cup (50 g) of shredded Italian blend cheese and the shredded Parmesan. Place the skillet on the top rack of the oven and let broil for 2 minutes, or until golden brown and bubbly. Serve family style.

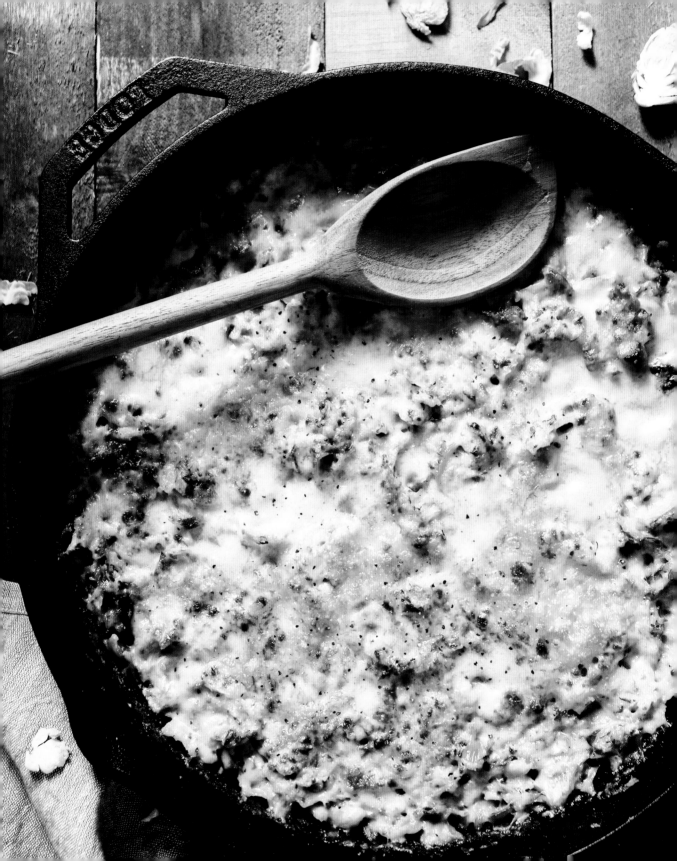

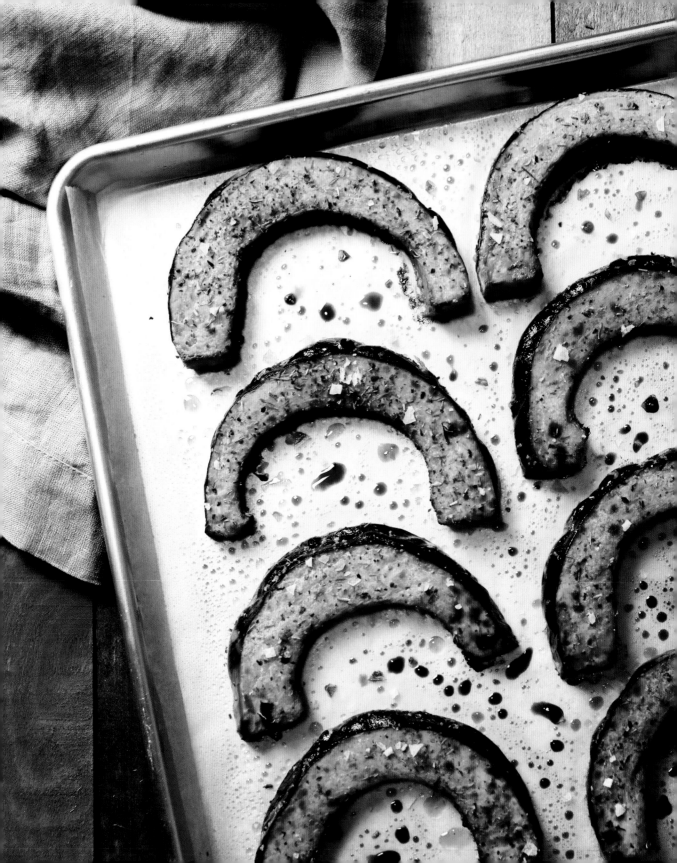

1 (3-lb [1.4-kg]) kabocha squash

3 tbsp (45 ml) olive oil

1½ tsp (9 g) kosher salt

2 tsp (12 g) herbes de Provence

1 tbsp (15 g) brown sugar alternative (optional)

½ tsp finishing flake salt

MACROS *per* SERVING

Calories: 97 • Fat: 6.9 g

Carbs: 9.3 g • Net Carbs: 7.3 g

Protein: 1.4 g

HERB-ROASTED KABOCHA SQUASH

Kabocha, also called Japanese pumpkin, is a really wonderful low-carb alternative to sweet potato, and tastes incredibly similar. Roasting the squash brings out all the wonderful flavors and the gorgeous bright orange color. And the herbs give it a wonderful floral note that complements the earthy, sweet flavor of the kabocha. You can find kabocha year-round at nearly any Asian market, but more and more you can now find it at many grocery stores, especially in the fall during pumpkin season. If you can't find it, butternut or acorn squash also work well in this recipe.

Try pairing this with the Secret-Recipe Whole Roasted Chicken (page 73).

Preheat your oven to 425°F (220°C). Line a baking sheet with aluminum foil. Cutting kabocha can be difficult, as the outer skin is very tough. Use a large, sharp knife to cut the squash in half from the stem to the root. Use a spoon to scoop out the seeds in the middle. Place the squash flat side down and cut it into ½-inch (1.3-cm) slices. Toss the squash in the olive oil to completely coat all sides. Place the slices on the prepared baking sheet.

Evenly coat both sides of the squash with the kosher salt and herbes de Provence. Then, sprinkle the top with the brown sugar alternative (if using) for a caramelized top. Bake for 30 minutes. Switch your oven to broil, move the baking sheet to the top rack of the oven and toast the squash for 5 minutes, or until golden brown. While still warm, sprinkle the finishing salt on top of the kabocha before serving.

1 lb (455 g) broccolini, dark green leaves removed

3 tbsp (45 ml) olive oil

1 tsp kosher salt

1½ tsp (8 ml) fresh lemon juice

MACROS *per* SERVING

Calories: 137 • Fat: 10.1 g

Carbs: 8.2 g • Net Carbs: 6.9 g

Protein: 4 g

LEMONY CHARRED BROCCOLINI

This gorgeous side dish is as tasty as it is beautiful. Charring the broccolini brings out the most wonderful smoky flavors. This easy recipe, finished really simply with a squeeze of lemon, yields truly spectacular results.

It's delicious paired with the Grilled Chicken Shawarma with Dill Yogurt Sauce (page 60).

Heat a cast-iron grill pan over high heat. You want the pan smoking hot. Meanwhile, in a large bowl, toss the broccolini with the olive oil and salt.

Once the pan is extremely hot, lay down the broccolini in one layer, so that the stems make full contact with the surface of the pan. You will likely need to cook the broccolini in two batches, as you do not want to overcrowd the pan. Cook the broccolini for 5 minutes. Do not stir or move the broccolini around in the pan. Just flip once halfway through. This will ensure beautiful grill marks. Keep the pan over high heat the entire time. You want to see smoke coming off the pan. Any broccolini with particularly thick stems may need an extra minute. Once cooked, place the broccolini on a long plate and drizzle with lemon juice before serving.

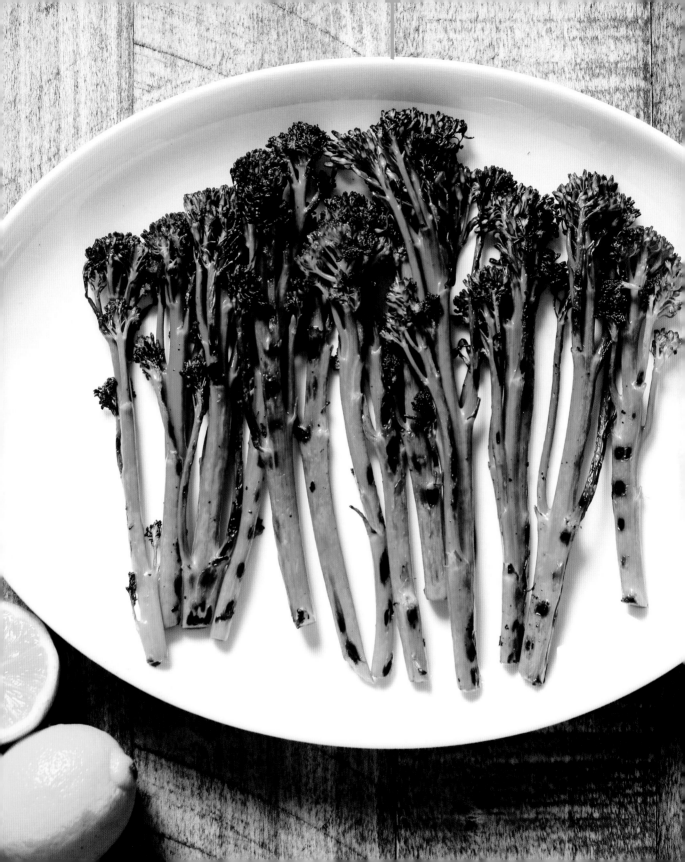

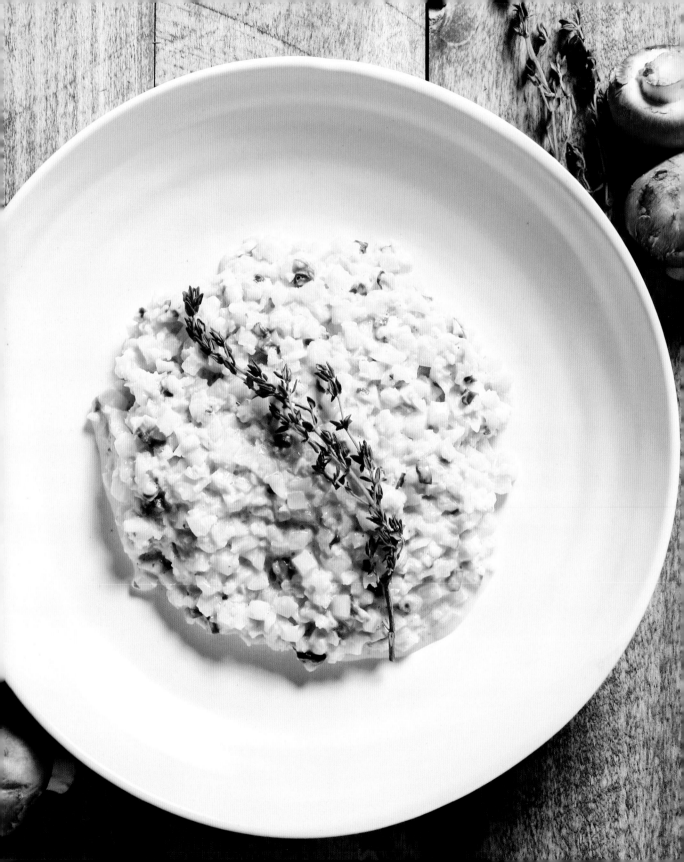

THE ULTIMATE CREAMY "RISOTTO"

This recipe is the epitome of decadence. The creamy and rich cauliflower risotto is the perfect side dish for nearly any dinner. What makes this recipe extra creamy is the crème fraîche. The mushrooms add umami and complexity to the dish, and of course, lots of Parmesan is absolutely necessary.

Try this with the Seared Ribeye with Blue Cheese & Chive Compound Butter (page 44).

In a large saucepan, heat the chicken stock over high heat. Bring it to a boil and reduce the stock until almost all the liquid has evaporated—this will take about 5 minutes. Then add 1 tablespoon (15 ml) of the olive oil, the finely chopped mushrooms and the garlic. Sauté the veggies for 2 minutes. Then add the cauliflower rice and remaining tablespoon (15 ml) of olive oil. Continue to sauté everything for about 4 minutes, or just until the cauliflower is cooked. The cauliflower should be al dente, not totally soft. Remove the pot from the heat and let cool slightly for about 5 minutes. Stir in the salt, crème fraîche, Parmesan and pepper. Spoon into a nice bowl and serve while hot.

2 tbsp (30 ml) avocado oil

3 tbsp (43 g) unsalted butter, divided

1 lb (455 g) button or cremini mushrooms, cut in half

3 cloves garlic, chopped

½ tsp kosher salt

¼ tsp freshly ground black pepper

¼ cup (60 ml) cognac or brandy

Chopped fresh parsley, for garnish (optional)

MACROS *per* SERVING

Calories: 208 • Fat: 14.2 g

Carbs: 7.5 g • Net Carbs: 6.5 g

Protein: 4 g

BUTTON MUSHROOM FLAMBÉ

If you want to put on a bit of a show, this is the recipe for you! The cognac does more than just create fire; it adds an incredibly deep flavor to the dish. This makes a great side dish for steak or chicken, and it's truly a fun way to create some sparks in your kitchen.

These go great with the Seared Ribeye with Blue Cheese & Chive Compound Butter (page 44).

Heat a large cast-iron pan over high heat. Once hot, add the avocado oil and 2 tablespoons (28 g) of the butter, then add the mushrooms, garlic, salt and pepper. Sauté for about 1 minute, stirring constantly.

Lower the heat to medium. Using an oven mitt to hold the handle of the pan, carefully pour in the cognac (do not pour directly from the bottle, as this is a fire hazard). Tilt the pan away from you and allow the alcohol to ignite. If you have an electric stove, use a long grill lighter to ignite the flame. Keep your hands and face away from the stove. The alcohol will burn off after just a few seconds. Add the remaining tablespoon (14 g) of butter and continue to sauté for another minute, just until the mushrooms are done. Serve in a nice bowl, garnished with chopped parsley (if using).

PRO TIP: Be very careful with open flame. Remove flammable objects from near the stove and keep a fire extinguisher nearby.

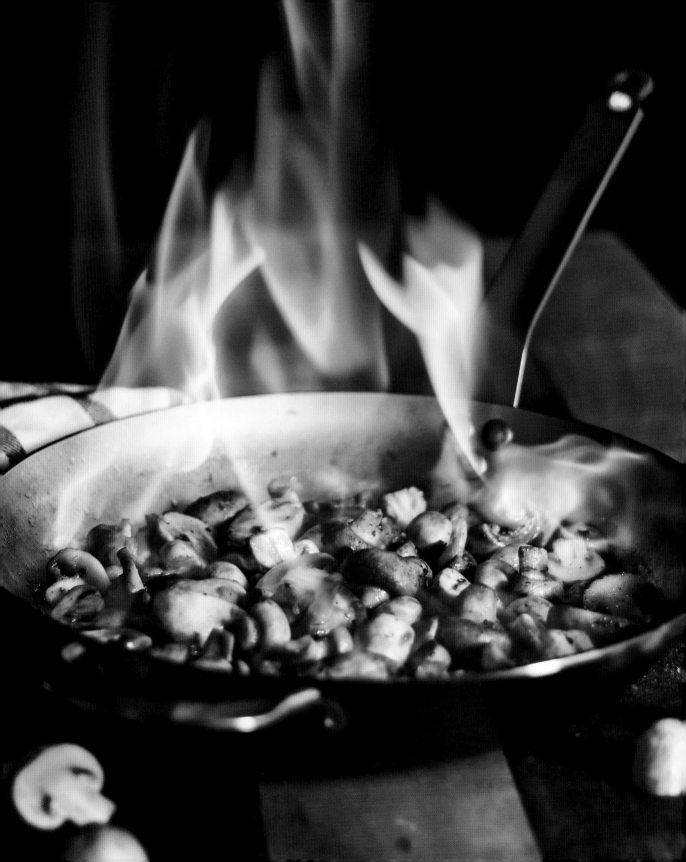

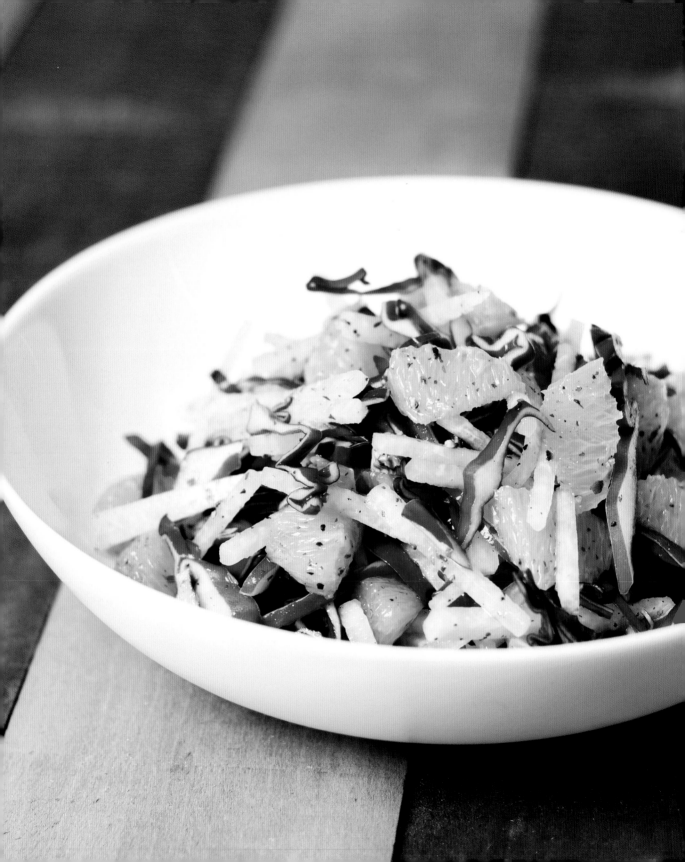

1 jicama

½ (2-lb [905-g]) head red cabbage

2 navel or Valencia oranges

½ cup (120 ml) cider vinegar
(I prefer Bragg organic)

½ tsp kosher salt

½ tsp freshly ground black pepper

½ tsp dried basil

1 tbsp (15 ml) extra virgin olive oil

MACROS *per* SERVING

Calories: 63 • Fat: 2.4 g

Carbs: 12.5 g • Net Carbs: 8.8 g

Protein: 1.4 g

JICAMA & ORANGE SLAW

This bright and colorful salad is a fantastic way to introduce jicama to your cooking. Jicama, a root vegetable native to Mexico, is delicious raw or cooked and has a surprisingly juicy and crisp center, reminiscent of an apple. Paired with the sweet orange slices and crunchy cabbage, this slaw hits all the right notes. Although jicama used to be harder to find, it's now readily available in most supermarkets across the country. I call this recipe a slaw, but it is nothing like the heavy, mayo-based coleslaws you may be used to, and it will be a nice talking point at your next cookout or picnic.

To make jicama matchsticks, cut the top and bottom off the jicama. Then, cut the four sides to create a peeled rectangular shape. Use a scale to check that you have 7 to 8 ounces (200 to 250 g) of peeled jicama. Then, cut it into very thin slices, about ⅛ inch (3 mm) thick. Lay the slices flat and cut them into matchsticks. Transfer them to a large bowl.

Remove the thick core from the half cabbage. Slice the cabbage down the middle, then very thinly shave the cabbage into slaw. Check that you have 10½ ounces (300 g) of shaved cabbage and add it to the bowl.

Next, make orange supremes: Slice off the top and bottom of the orange. Then, run the knife along the outside of the orange to remove all the peel and pith, avoiding the flesh. Once you have a clean, "naked" orange, use the knife to cut each orange segment from its surrounding membrane, to create perfect orange segments. Once you've removed all the orange wedges, squeeze the remaining orange into the bowl, as we wouldn't want to waste all that delicious juice. Slice the orange segments in half and place them in the bowl of jicama.

Add the vinegar, salt, pepper, basil and olive oil, and stir well. Let the slaw rest in the fridge for 30 minutes to an hour to marinate. Stir again before serving.

SWEET TREATS

LOOK, WE ALL KNOW THAT NO MEAL IS TRULY complete without dessert. However, without sugar and flour, desserts can sometimes be frustrating. But not this time. These sweet treats are so decadent, you'll forget they are Keto!

Berry Cheesecake Trifle (page 116)

Spiced Carrot Cake with Cardamom Cream Cheese Frosting (page 119)

Caramel Flan with Candy Tuile (page 120)

Strawberry Balsamic Ice Cream (page 123)

Key Lime Cheesecake (page 124)

Fluffy "Churro" Donuts (page 127)

Chocolate Peanut Butter Pie (page 128)

Buttery Ghee Pound Cake (page 131)

Tres Leches Cupcakes with Cinnamon Whipped Frosting (page 132)

Tiramisu Mousse (page 135)

1 lb (455 g) strawberries, hulled
and cut in half, divided

12 oz (340 g) raspberries, divided

12 oz (340 g) blackberries,
divided

6 oz (170 g) blueberries, divided

1½ cups (294 g) allulose or
erythritol sweetener, divided

1½ lb (680 g) cream cheese, at
room temperature

1 pint (475 ml) heavy whipping
cream

Fresh mint leaves, for garnish
(optional)

MACROS *per* SERVING

Calories: 382 • Fat: 33.3 g

Carbs: 13.4 g • Net Carbs: 9.3 g

Protein: 5.9 g

BERRY CHEESECAKE TRIFLE

This no-bake dessert is definitely a showstopper. The layered trifle is packed with the flavors of summer, and the salty cheesecake layer balances the sweet berries. Make this for your next family holiday, and your guests won't even notice it's Keto.

In a small saucepan, combine half of the strawberries, raspberries, blackberries and blueberries with 1 cup (196 g) of sweetener. Heat over low heat, stirring occasionally, just until the berries are soft. Pour them into a bowl and place it in the freezer for a few minutes to cool.

In a bowl, using a spatula or hand mixer, beat the cream cheese until fluffy, then set aside. Once the berry mixture is cooled, add it to the cream cheese and mix it together until well combined. Next, using a stand mixer with the whisk attachment or a hand mixer, make the whipped cream by combining the remaining ½ cup (98 g) of sweetener with the cream and beating until stiff peaks are formed.

Assemble the trifle: Start with a layer of the berry cream cheese mixture, then add a layer of whipped cream, then top with a combination of the remaining fresh berries. Repeat until you have three layers of each component. Top with a little more whipped cream and a few fresh mint leaves (if using). Place in the fridge to set for at least 2 hours or overnight before serving.

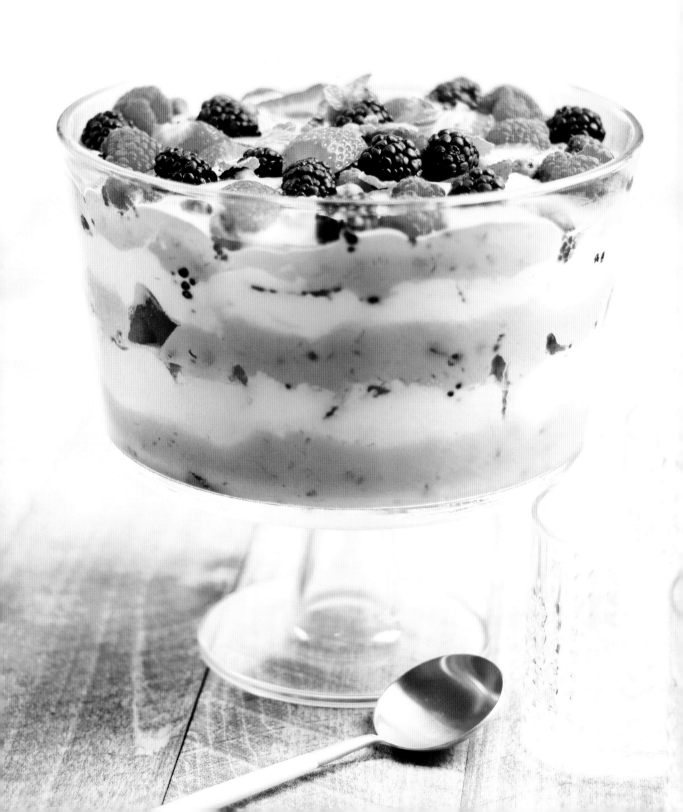

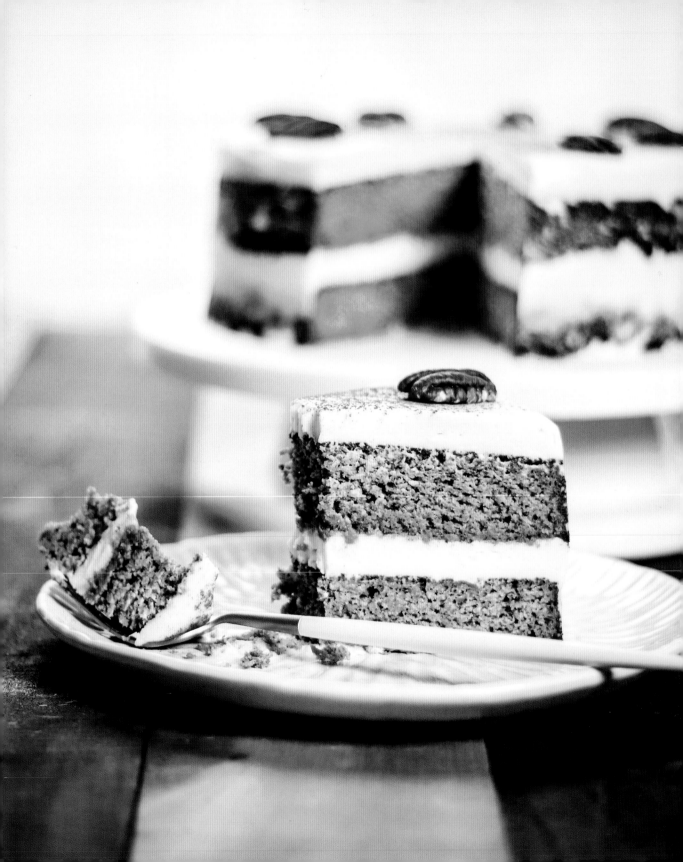

SPICED CARROT CAKE

Nonstick cooking spray

3 cups (300 g) almond flour

1½ cups (294 g) allulose sweetener

2 tsp (9 g) baking powder

3 tbsp (21 g) ground cinnamon

2 tsp (4 g) ground cloves

2 tsp (4 g) ground ginger

1 tsp ground nutmeg

1 tsp ground coriander

1 tsp ground cardamom

¼ tsp kosher salt

1 cup (225 g or 2 sticks) unsalted
butter, melted

4 large eggs

½ cup (230 g) sour cream

2 cups (270 g) shredded carrot

FROSTING

1½ lb (680 g) cream cheese, at room
temperature

1½ cups (337 g or 3 sticks) unsalted
butter, at room temperature

1 cup (192 g) allulose sweetener

1½ tsp (3 g) ground cardamom

¼ tsp vanilla extract

¼ tsp kosher salt

8 to 10 pecan halves, for garnish

Ground cinnamon, for garnish

SPICED CARROT CAKE WITH CARDAMOM CREAM CHEESE FROSTING

While I was growing up, my mother made the most wonderful carrot cakes for our birthdays. The cream cheese frosting was (and still is) my favorite part, so I decided to make a Keto version. And after traveling through India and being completely inspired by the vast spice markets, I thought I would try something new by adding some warm spices to both the cake and the frosting, for an extra-special punch of flavor.

Prepare the cake: Preheat your oven to 350°F (180°C). Spray two 9-inch (23-cm) round cake pans with cooking spray. In a large bowl, combine the almond flour, allulose, baking powder, cinnamon, cloves, ginger, nutmeg, coriander, cardamom and salt. Mix well. Then, mix in the melted butter, eggs and sour cream. Finally, add the shredded carrot and mix until just combined. Divide the batter evenly between the cake pans. Bake for 25 minutes. Remove the cakes from the oven and let them cool completely in the pan.

Meanwhile, make the cream cheese frosting: In the bowl of a stand mixer fitted with the whisk attachment, combine the softened cream cheese and butter. Beat for 2 to 3 minutes, or until light and fluffy. Then, add the allulose, cardamom, vanilla and salt. Beat for another 2 minutes, or until the frosting is completely smooth.

Once the cakes are completely cool, spread half of the frosting on top of the first layer. Stack the second cake on top, then add the second half of the frosting. Spread the frosting evenly and top with pecan halves and a sprinkle of cinnamon, then serve.

MACROS *per* SERVING

Calories: 767 • Fat: 75.1 g • Carbs: 10.3 g •
Net Carbs: 6.6 g • Protein: 12.9 g

Nonstick cooking spray

1½ cups (294 g) allulose
sweetener, divided

2 tbsp (30 ml) water

2 cups (475 ml) heavy whipping
cream

1½ tsp (8 ml) vanilla extract

2 large eggs

2 large egg yolks

MACROS *per* SERVING

Calories: 480 • Fat: 49.7 g

Carbs: 3.9 g • Net Carbs: 3.9 g

Protein: 6.6 g

CARAMEL FLAN WITH CANDY TUILE

There is nothing like flan. The creamy custard bakes with the rich caramel and creates sweet perfection, and the candy "sugar art" is guaranteed to impress. Note: You must use allulose for this recipe, or the caramelization will not be the same.

Preheat the oven to 325°F (170°C). Lightly spray four 8-ounce (240-ml) ramekins with cooking spray and place them in a single layer in a casserole or baking dish.

Make the caramel: In a small saucepan, combine 1 cup (196 g) of the allulose and the water. Place the pot over medium-high heat. Without stirring, the allulose will dissolve and the liquid will start to bubble. Keep an eye on the pot, as the liquid will turn from clear to yellow to brown. Once it gets brown and you can no longer see the bottom of the pan, immediately remove the pan from the heat. Divide the caramel equally among the four ramekins.

In another saucepan over medium heat, heat the cream, vanilla and the remaining ½ cup (98 g) of allulose until the mixture reaches 165°F (73°C). If you don't have a thermometer, heat it just until you start to see a little steam, but do not boil. Then, in a bowl, whisk together the 2 eggs plus the 2 yolks. While whisking constantly, very slowly add a splash of the cream mixture to the eggs. Continue to add the cream mixture to the eggs as you whisk—be sure to do this extremely slowly or you will scramble the eggs. Once everything is combined, divide the mixture equally among the ramekins. Ensuring no water splashes inside the ramekins, add very hot tap water to the casserole dish, enough to reach halfway up the outer sides of the ramekins. Carefully place the dish in the oven, then bake for 50 minutes without opening the oven door. Remove the ramekins from the hot water bath and let them cool for 15 minutes. Use a small knife to cut around the edge of the flans, to make sure they don't stick, and then flip them over onto a plate to unmold.

You will need a silicone mat or parchment paper to make the candy tuile. Take an unmolded ramekin with the remaining caramel still stuck inside. Microwave it at full power for 20 seconds. Let the caramel cool and thicken slightly, then drizzle it over the silicone mat in a random swirl pattern. Repeat with the other ramekins. Once the swirls cool and harden, you will be able to peel them off the mat and use them as a beautiful garnish. Serve the flans warm or cold.

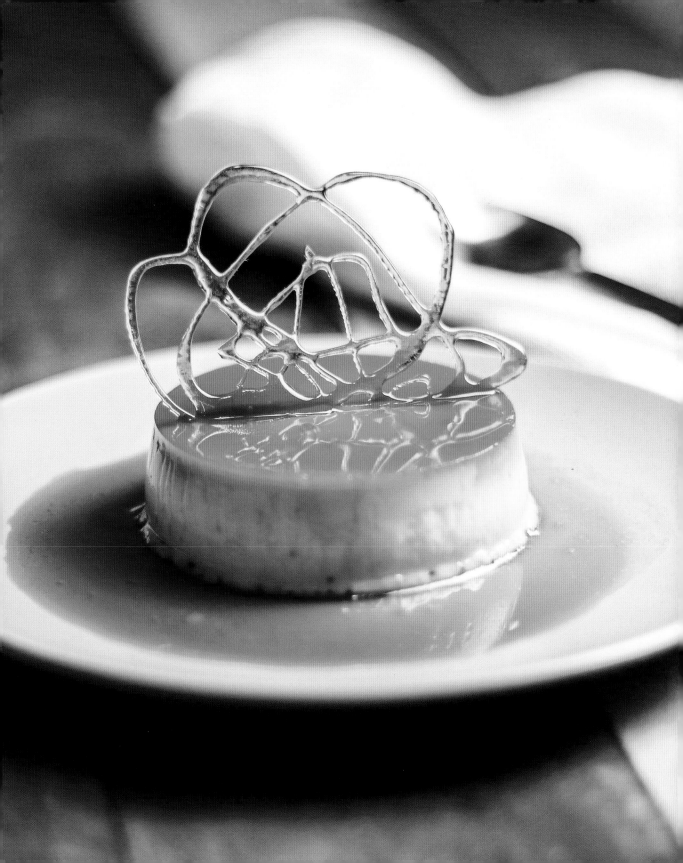

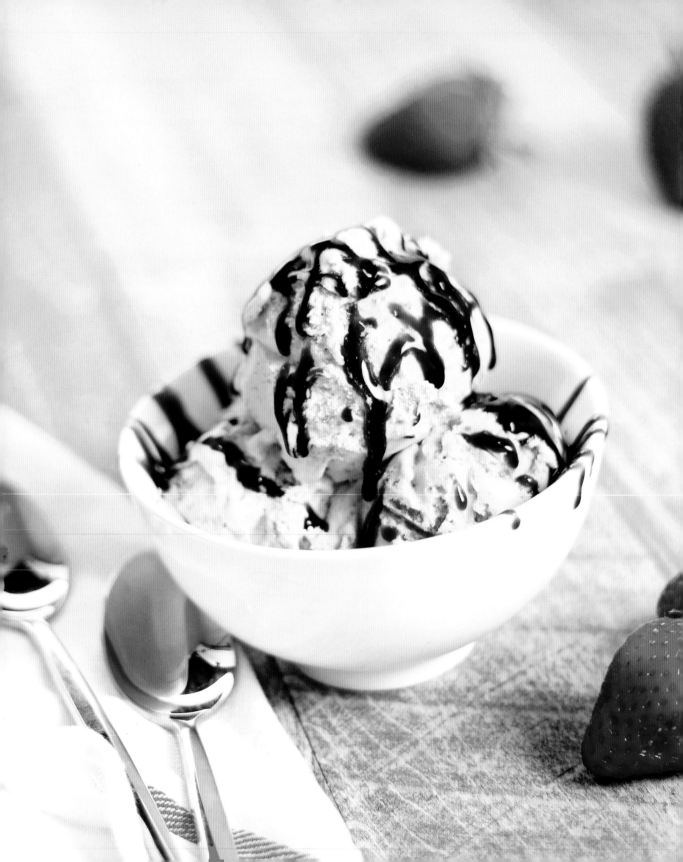

3 cups (710 ml) heavy whipping cream

1 cup (192 g) allulose sweetener

¼ tsp xanthan gum

2 tsp (10 ml) vanilla extract

1 lb (455 g) strawberries

3 tbsp (45 ml) balsamic vinegar

Aged balsamic vinegar, or Homemade Balsamic Reduction (page 77), for drizzling (optional)

MACROS *per* SERVING

Calories: 334 • Fat: 33.5 g

Carbs: 7.9 g • Net Carbs: 6.8 g

Protein: 2.3 g

STRAWBERRY BALSAMIC ICE CREAM

This twist on a classic brings this summery treat to new heights. The strawberries provide natural sweetness and color, while the balsamic vinegar brings the perfect tangy complexity to this must-try ice cream. The best part is, it only has six ingredients. With this recipe, you must use allulose as the sweetener, to prevent the ice cream from crystallizing.

In a saucepan, heat the cream, allulose, xanthan gum and vanilla over medium-high heat. Whisk aggressively until everything is dissolved, but do not bring to a boil. Pour the mixture into a bowl and place it in the fridge to cool down completely.

Meanwhile, cut the strawberries into roughly ½-inch (1.3-cm) cubes (no need for perfection). Add the strawberries to a saucepan along with the balsamic vinegar. Bring it to a boil, then lower the heat to low and cook for 15 minutes. This will reduce the mixture to a syrupy consistency. Place the syrup in the fridge to cool completely.

Once everything is chilled, you can pour the cream mixture and strawberry syrup into your ice-cream maker. Run the ice-cream maker according to the manufacturer's directions (my Cuisinart takes 20 minutes). You can eat the ice cream immediately after (almost like soft-serve), or place it in the freezer to set into firm ice cream. Serve with a light drizzle of aged balsamic vinegar on top (if using) or your own sugar-free homemade balsamic reduction.

"GRAHAM" CRUST

Nonstick cooking spray

2 cups (200 g) almond flour

2 tbsp (15 g) coconut flour

¼ cup (48 g) allulose sweetener

2 tsp (6 g) ground cinnamon

¼ tsp kosher salt

6 tbsp (84 g or ¾ stick) unsalted
butter, melted

KEY LIME CHEESECAKE

3 lb (1.4 kg) cream cheese, at
room temperature

6 large eggs

½ cup (115 g) sour cream

1½ cups (294 g) allulose
sweetener

1 tsp vanilla extract

½ tsp kosher salt

¾ cup (175 ml) fresh Key lime
juice (from about 1 lb [455 g]
Key limes)

6 cups (1.4 L) boiling water

Fresh whipped cream, shredded
coconut, or Key lime slices, for
garnish (optional)

MACROS *per* SERVING

Calories: 632 • Fat: 56.6 g

Carbs: 10.2 g • Net Carbs: 7.7 g

Protein: 15.4 g

KEY LIME CHEESECAKE

Key lime pie and cheesecake are two of the truly great American desserts, and something magical happens when you combine them. The tart lime balances the rich and creamy cheesecake to create the most stunning summery treat. Best of all, this is totally Keto-friendly, with none of the added sugars. Hopefully, you can find Key limes in your grocery store, but if not, regular limes will still do the trick.

Prepare the crust: Preheat your oven to 325°F (170°C). Spray the sides and bottom of a 9-inch (23-cm) springform pan with cooking spray. Then, trace the outline of the pan on parchment paper, cut out the circle and press the parchment into the bottom of the pan (the oil will help the paper stick to the pan). Wrap the outside bottom of the pan with aluminum foil, ensuring the foil wraps up the sides, to prevent leaks.

In a bowl, combine the almond flour, coconut flour, allulose, cinnamon, salt and melted butter. Mix well with a fork until it looks like wet sand. Press the mixture into the bottom of the springform pan to form an even layer. Poke the bottom several times with a fork, then bake for 20 minutes. Remove from the oven and set the pan aside to cool.

Prepare the cheesecake: In the bowl of a stand mixer fitted with the paddle attachment (or using a hand mixer with a large bowl), whip the softened cream cheese for at least 1 minute, or until fluffy. With the mixer running on low speed, add the eggs, one at a time, then add the sour cream, allulose, vanilla, salt and Key lime juice, and mix until the mixture is smooth.

Pour the cream cheese mixture over the crust in the springform pan (make sure the crust has cooled first). Place the springform pan on a rimmed cookie sheet and transfer the pan and sheet together to the middle rack of the oven. Carefully pour the boiling water into the cookie sheet, taking care not to pour any water into the springform pan. Bake for exactly 75 minutes without opening the oven door (the steam is important). Then, turn off the oven and leave the cake inside with the oven door closed for 30 minutes. Crack open the oven door and let cool slowly for another 30 minutes. Remove the cheesecake from the oven and place it in the fridge to cool overnight.

Garnish with fresh simple whipped cream, shredded coconut or thin slices of Key lime (if using).

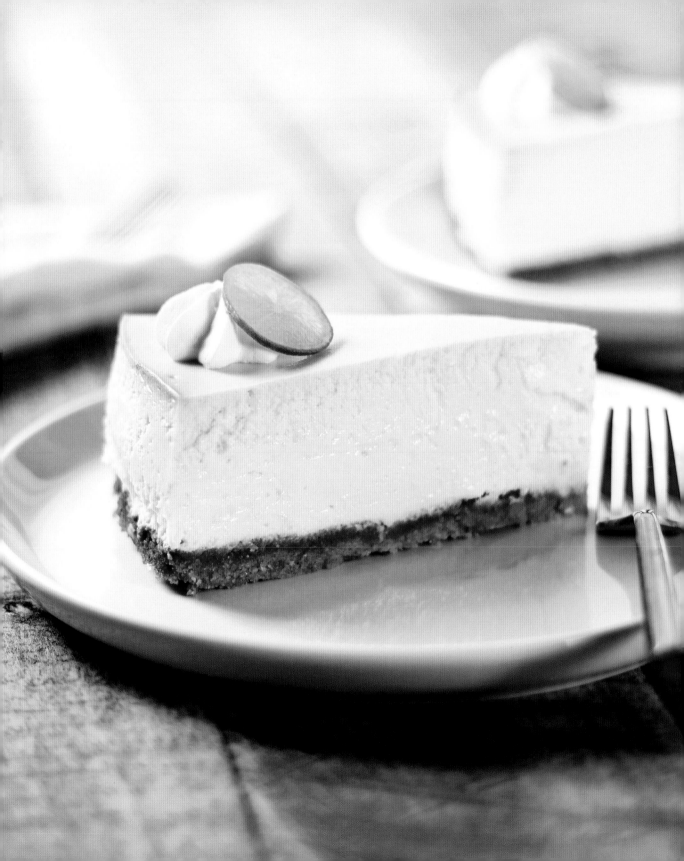

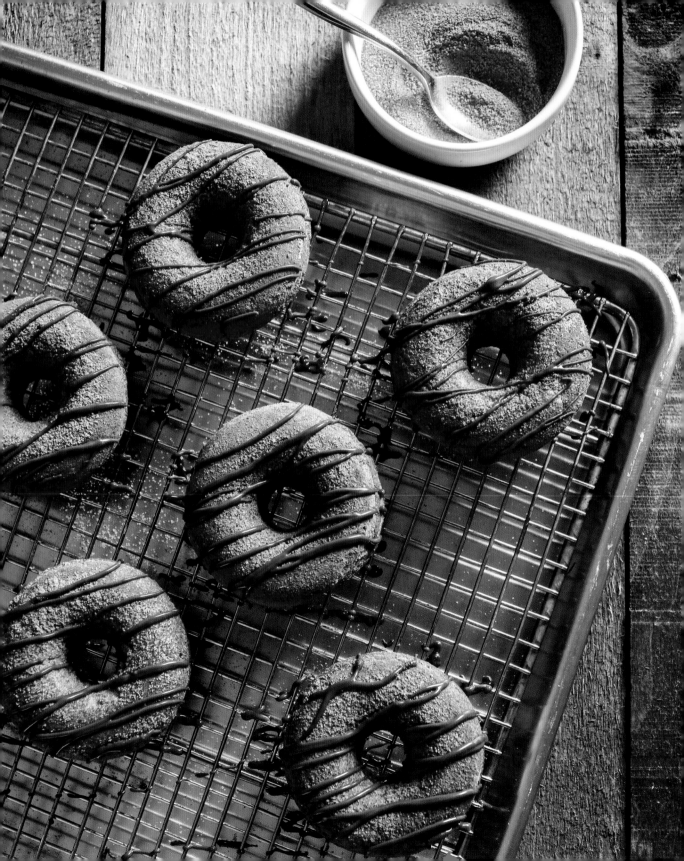

DONUTS

2 large eggs

¾ cup (75 g) almond flour

½ cup (96 g) allulose or erythritol
sweetener

3 tbsp (45 ml) heavy whipping
cream

1 tsp vanilla extract

½ tsp baking powder

½ tsp xanthan gum

½ tsp ground cinnamon

CINNAMON SUGAR COATING

¼ cup (48 g) granulated erythritol
or allulose

3 tbsp (21 g) ground cinnamon

2 oz (55 g) sugar-free dark
chocolate or baker's chocolate
(chips or bars)

MACROS *per* SERVING

Calories: 194 ● Fat: 17.8 g

Carbs: 6.8 g ● Net Carbs: 3.1 g

Protein: 6.3 g

FLUFFY "CHURRO" DONUTS

There are few things I love as much as a good donut, and this fun (and healthier) version brings the sweet cinnamon flavors of churros, the Mexican street food staple, right to your kitchen. Drizzled with warm chocolate, these are the ultimate dessert (though you must try dipping them in your morning coffee, too).

Prepare the donuts: Preheat your oven to 400°F (200°C). Use a food processor (or immersion blender and a bowl) to blend all of the donut ingredients until very smooth. Pour evenly into the six wells of a greased silicone donut mold (you can easily find inexpensive molds in cookware shops or on Amazon). Set the silicone mold on a cookie sheet (for stability) and place the pan in the oven to bake for 15 minutes. Remove from the oven and let cool.

While the donuts cool, prepare the cinnamon sugar coating: On a shallow plate, combine the sweetener and cinnamon. Once cool enough to handle, remove the donuts from the molds and toss them in the cinnamon sugar coating.

Place the chocolate (broken into smaller pieces, if not chips) in a microwave-safe bowl. Microwave on full power for 30 seconds, stir and repeat until the chocolate is smooth and melted. Use a spoon to drizzle the chocolate on top of the donuts.

PIE CRUST

2 cups (200 g) almond flour

2 tbsp (15 g) coconut flour

¼ cup (48 g) allulose sweetener

1 tsp ground cinnamon

½ tsp kosher salt

6 tbsp (84 g or ¾ stick) unsalted butter, melted

CHOCOLATE PEANUT BUTTER FILLING

1½ cups (294 g) allulose sweetener

¼ cup (28 g) unsweetened cacao powder

¼ tsp kosher salt

2 large eggs

¾ cup (175 ml) heavy whipping cream

6 tbsp (96 g) natural, no-sugar added, smooth peanut butter, divided

Fresh whipped cream, for garnish (optional)

MACROS *per* SERVING

Calories: 428 • Fat: 40 g

Carbs: 11.2 g • Net Carbs: 5.7 g

Protein: 11.4 g

CHOCOLATE PEANUT BUTTER PIE

This twist on a chocolate pie has all the flavors of a peanut butter cup, but without any of the sugar. The chocolate custard filling is so silky and smooth, and the crumb crust is perfectly salty. But what makes this pie even more special is the peanut butter swirl marbled on top. Yum!

Prepare the crust: Preheat your oven to 350°F (180°C). In a bowl, combine all the pie crust ingredients until they achieve a wet-sand consistency. Using your fingers, evenly press the crust into the bottom and sides of an 8-inch (20-cm) pie pan. Then, use aluminum foil to make a "collar" around the crust, to prevent burning. Set the pan aside.

Prepare the filling: In a large bowl, stir together the allulose, cacao powder and salt. Mix well, then add the eggs, cream and 2 tablespoons (32 g) of the peanut butter. Stir well to completely combine the mixture. Pour over the pie crust in its pan.

In a small microwave-safe bowl, heat the remaining ¼ cup (64 g) of peanut butter for 15 to 30 seconds in a microwave on full power, then drizzle the warm peanut butter on the top of the pie in a spiral design. Use a skewer or toothpick to "marble" the peanut butter swirl.

Bake the pie for 50 minutes. The center of the pie will still be slightly jiggly. Remove from the oven and let cool for at least 2 hours, or until completely cool. Store it in the fridge, and serve it with some fresh whipped cream (if using).

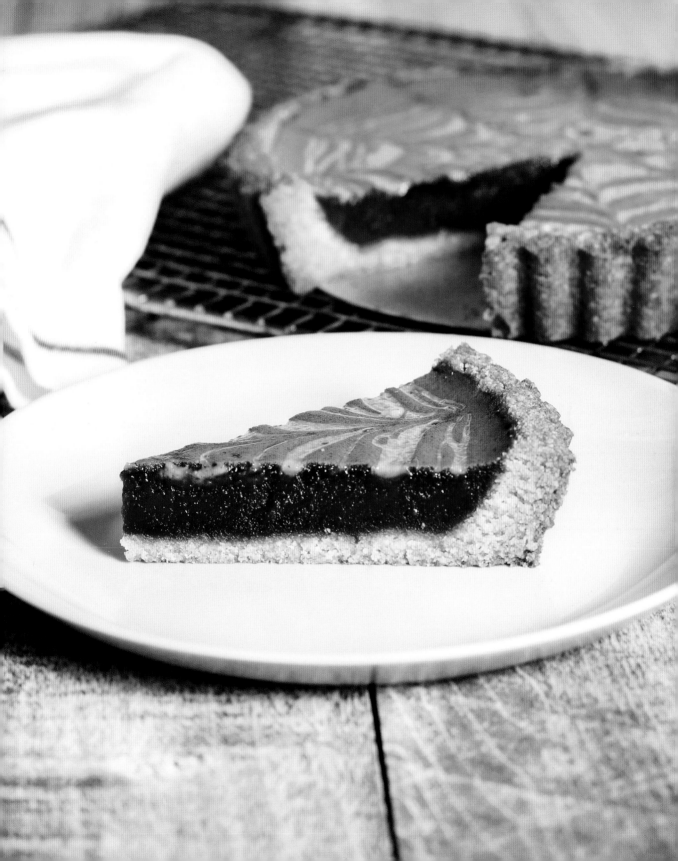

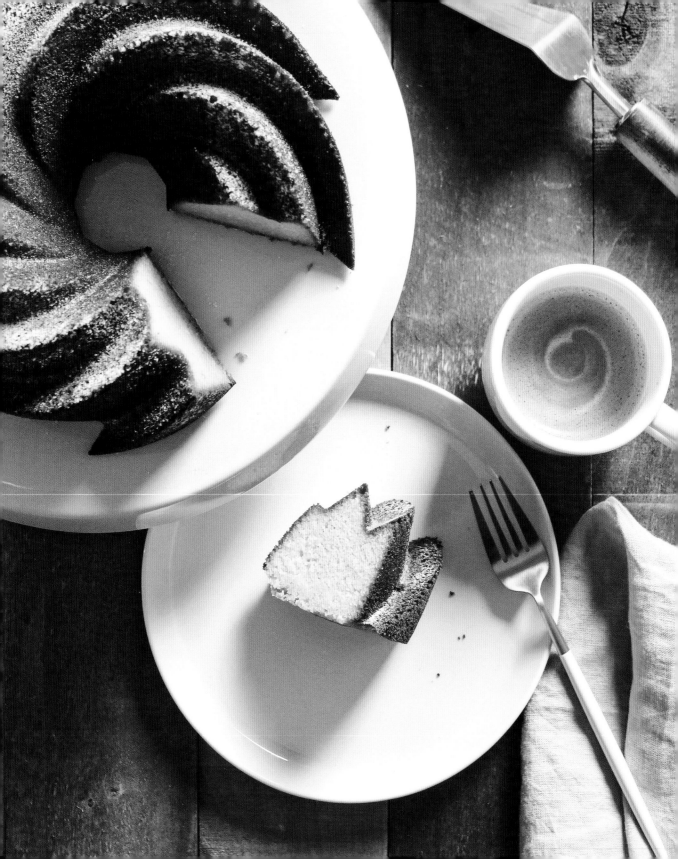

Nonstick cooking spray

⅓ cup (75 g) ghee, melted

4 oz (115 g) cream cheese, at room
temperature

5 large eggs, at room temperature

¼ cup (60 ml) heavy cream

1 tbsp (15 ml) vanilla extract

1½ tsp (7 ml) almond extract

1½ tsp (7 ml) butter extract

1½ cups (150 g) almond flour

⅓ cup (35 g) coconut flour

1 cup (192 g) allulose sweetener

½ tsp baking powder

⅛ tsp kosher salt

MACROS *per* SERVING

Calories: 334 • Fat: 32.2 g

Carbs: 5.2 g • Net Carbs: 2.6 g

Protein: 6.5 g

BUTTERY GHEE POUND CAKE

Ghee, also known as clarified butter, is used throughout India and much of the Middle East. It has way more flavor than butter, and gives this pound cake an extra-buttery note. This is one of those dishes where you just can't tell it's Keto. It's just that damn good. It's absolutely perfect for dessert, or for breakfast with a cup of your favorite coffee.

Preheat your oven to 350°F (180°C). Grease a 10-inch (25-cm) Bundt pan with nonstick spray.

In a small, microwave-safe bowl, melt the ghee in a microwave. In another microwave-safe bowl, heat the cream cheese in the microwave on full power for 30 seconds until it's warm and soft. In a large bowl, combine the eggs, cream, extracts, ghee and cream cheese. Use a hand mixer to combine the ingredients extremely well. Be sure the mixture is totally blended; you do not want lumps of cream cheese. Add the almond flour, coconut flour, sweetener, baking powder and salt. Using a spatula, mix until just combined. Pour the batter into the prepared pan. Bake for 30 to 40 minutes, or until a wooden skewer inserted into the center comes out clean.

Remove the cake from the oven and let it cool completely before removing from the pan. Once cool to the touch, carefully flip the pan onto a plate or cake stand to release the cake, and serve.

COCONUT TRES LECHES CUPCAKES

1 cup (112 g) coconut flour

½ cup plus 2 tbsp (126 g) allulose sweetener, divided

2 tsp (10 g) baking powder

1 tsp ground cinnamon

¼ tsp kosher salt

4 tbsp (57 g or ½ stick) unsalted butter, melted

4 large eggs

1 cup (230 g) sour cream

1 tbsp (15 ml) vanilla extract

¾ cup (175 ml) heavy whipping cream

CINNAMON WHIPPED CREAM FROSTING

1 cup (240 ml) heavy whipping cream

¼ cup (48 g) allulose sweetener

½ tsp vanilla extract

½ tsp ground cinnamon, plus more for dusting

MACROS *per* SERVING

Calories: 236 • Fat: 21.5 g

Carbs: 8.1 g • Net Carbs: 4.6 g

Protein: 2.8 g

TRES LECHES CUPCAKES WITH CINNAMON WHIPPED FROSTING

Tres leches cake (meaning "three milk" cake in Spanish) is the quintessential Latin American dessert, and every time I take a bite, I'm transported right back to Mexico. What makes this cake so unique is that it's soaked in milk to make it supermoist. Every Latin household has their own recipe, and may argue as to the origins of tres leches, or exactly how to make it. But this is my Keto version, miniaturized into cupcakes. There is sour cream in the cake batter (milk #1), cream to soak the cake (#2) and whipped cream on top (#3).

Prepare the cupcakes: Preheat your oven to 350°F (180°C). Line a twelve-well cupcake pan with cupcake liners.

In a large bowl, combine the coconut flour, ½ cup (96 g) of allulose, baking powder, cinnamon and salt. Mix well. Then, add the melted butter, eggs, sour cream and vanilla. Mix well. Evenly divide the batter among the twelve cupcake liners. Bake for 25 minutes, then remove from the oven and let the cupcakes cool completely in the pan for at least 1 hour.

Using a skewer or chopstick, poke several holes in the top of the cupcakes. In a small bowl, mix together the cream and remaining 2 tablespoons (30 g) of allulose. Very slowly pour 2 teaspoons (10 ml) of the cream mixture into each cupcake.

Prepare the frosting: In the bowl of a stand mixer fitted with the whisk attachment, combine the heavy cream and allulose. Whip on high speed until very stiff peaks form. Add the vanilla and cinnamon, and whip for another 10 to 15 seconds. Use a piping bag to decorate the cupcakes. Dust the top with more cinnamon, and store the cupcakes in the fridge in an airtight container.

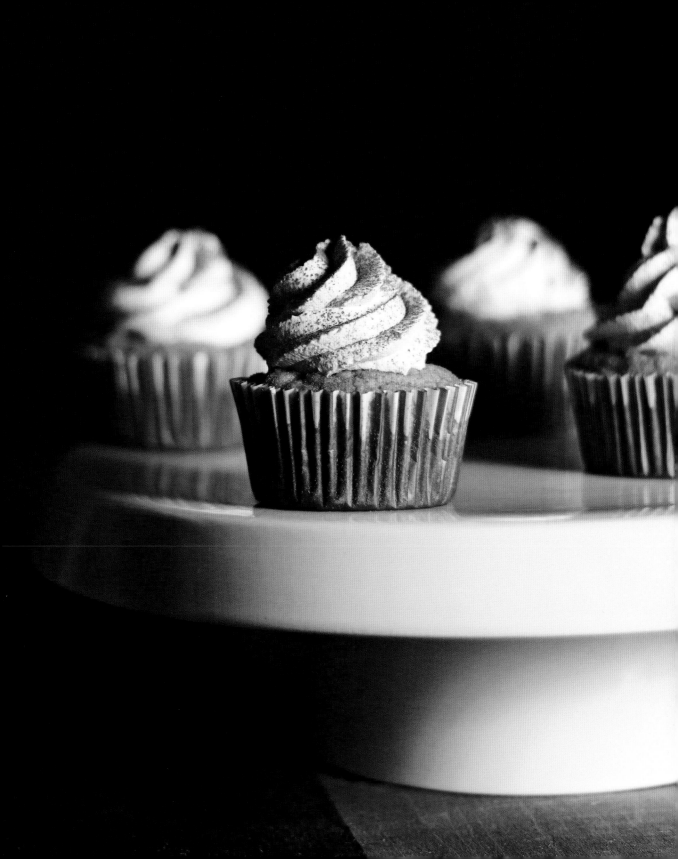

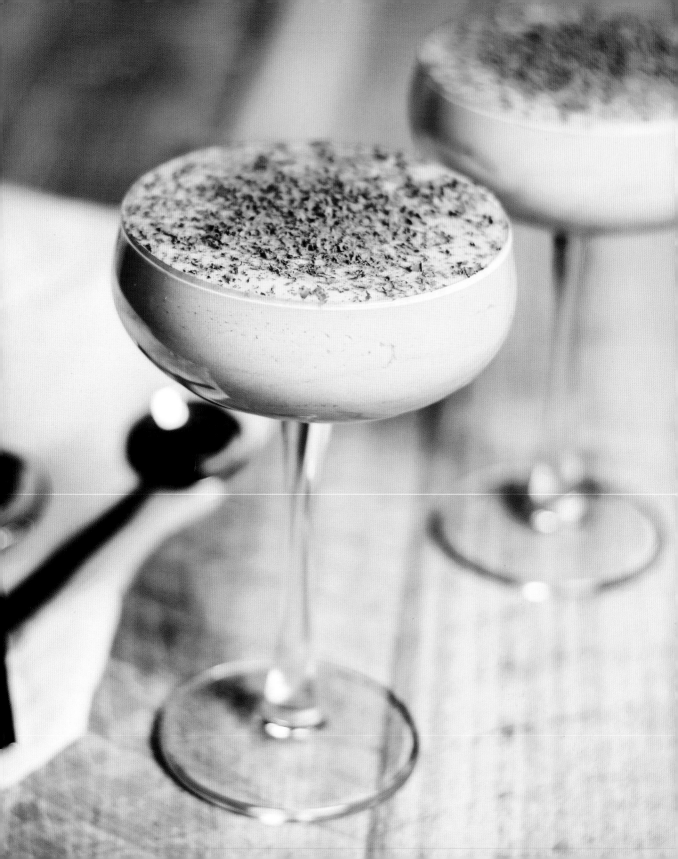

MAKES FOUR 6-OZ (170-G) PORTIONS

¼ cup (20 g) instant espresso powder

1 tbsp (15 ml) hot water

1 lb (455 g) cold mascarpone cheese (see Pro Tip)

1 cup (240 ml) cold heavy whipping cream (see Pro Tip)

½ cup (96 g) allulose sweetener

½ tsp vanilla extract

⅛ tsp ground cinnamon, plus more for garnish

½ oz (14 g) sugar-free dark chocolate or baker's 100% chocolate

MACROS *per* SERVING

Calories: 722 • Fat: 76 g

Carbs: 4.8 g • Net Carbs: 4.3 g

Protein: 9.7 g

TIRAMISU MOUSSE

The classic Italian tiramisu is made simple here. This sugar-free, no-bake dessert is so easy, and yet so beautiful. The coffee flavor pairs perfectly with the light saltiness from the mascarpone. It's also perfect for a dinner party, since you can make it ahead and leave it in the fridge (in fact, it only gets better overnight in the fridge).

In a small bowl, combine the instant espresso and hot water, stir to dissolve the espresso, then set aside.

In a stand mixer fitted with the whisk attachment, whip the cold mascarpone on high speed for 30 seconds, or until fluffy. Stop the mixer and add the cream. Turn on the mixer, starting at low speed and gradually increasing to high speed, and whip until stiff peaks are formed. Add the allulose, vanilla and cinnamon, and whip on high speed for another 30 seconds, scraping down the sides of the bowl as needed.

To serve, spoon the mousse into cups (or use a piping bag). Use a microplane or grater to shave the chocolate over the top. Add a light dusting of cinnamon, and place the cups in the fridge to cool for at least 1 hour. You can also make these a day or two ahead and leave them in the fridge.

PRO TIP: Leave the mascarpone and heavy cream in the fridge until right before using—you want them to stay cold for this recipe.

EASY SAUCES
& MARINADES

I FIRMLY BELIEVE THAT A GOOD SAUCE CAN TAKE a simple meal and make it special. These sauces are bold and flavorful and can be paired with almost any protein, such as steak, chicken or fish, to create something beautiful for your kitchen table. Many of the sauces double as

Spicy Red Chimichurri (page 138)

Garlic Aioli (The Best Mayo from Scratch) (page 141)

Avocado Salsa Verde (page 142)

Secret-Ingredient Cheese Sauce (page 145)

Meyer Lemon Vinaigrette (page 146)

Easy Tahini Yogurt Sauce (page 149)

Japanese Sesame Ginger Dressing (page 150)

Zesty Dill Rémoulade (page 153)

Cinnamon Caramel Sauce (page 154)

3 canned chipotle peppers in
adobo (scant 2 oz [50 g])

½ cup packed (20 g) fresh
cilantro

⅓ cup (80 ml) olive oil

1 tsp paprika

5 cloves garlic

3 tbsp (45 ml) cider vinegar
(I prefer Bragg organic)

½ tsp kosher salt

MACROS *per* SERVING (2 TBSP [30 ML])

Calories: 174 • Fat: 18.3 g

Carbs: 3.2 g • Net Carbs: 2.7 g

Protein: 0.4 g

SPICY RED CHIMICHURRI

I'm sure you've had a classic green chimichurri, but this spicy red version may surprise you, and it goes surprisingly well with just about any meat. You can use it as a marinade, or as a sauce to drizzle on steak or roasted chicken. The chipotle peppers give it a smokiness and complexity that really heightens anything it touches, such as the Secret-Recipe Whole Roasted Chicken (page 73).

Use a fork to remove the individual peppers from the can and place them in a food processor along with all the other ingredients. Blend for about 60 seconds, or until combined. Store it in a jar, and save it in your fridge for up to a week.

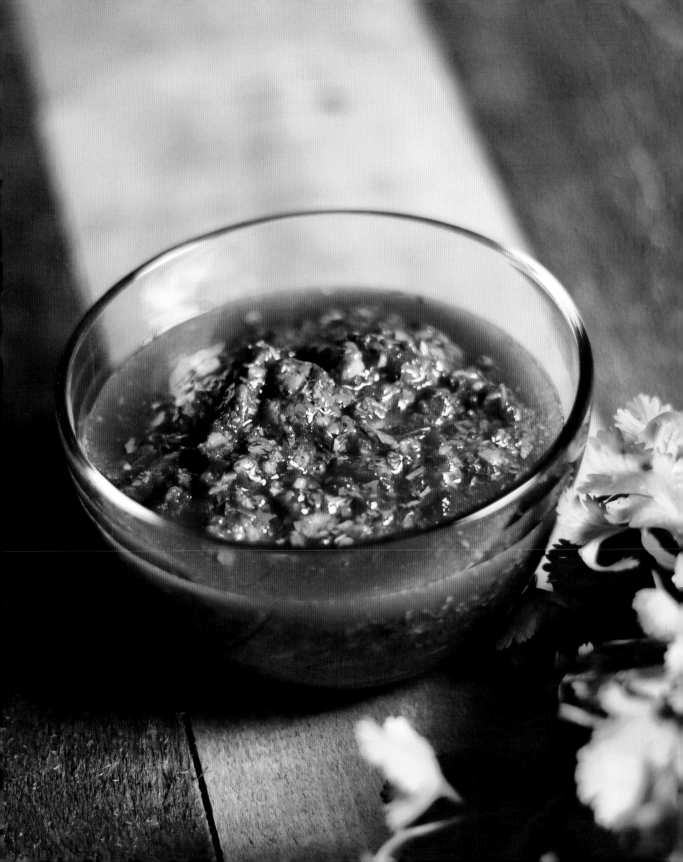

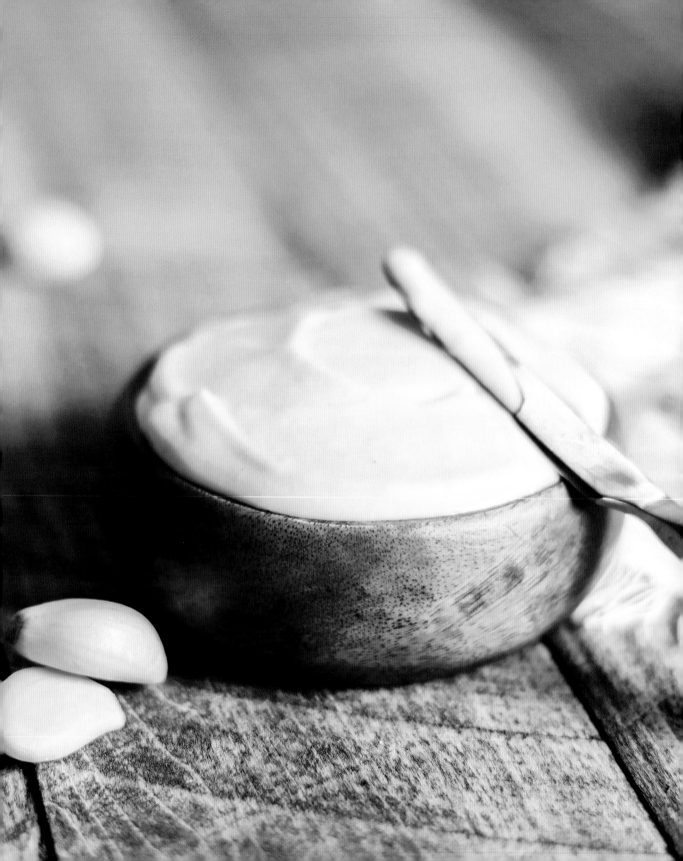

1 large clove garlic

1 cup (240 ml) avocado oil

1 tbsp (11 g) Dijon mustard

½ tsp kosher salt

1 large egg

MACROS *per* SERVING (2 TBSP [30 ML])

Calories: 260 • Fat: 28.8 g

Carbs: 0.3 g • Net Carbs: 0.3 g

Protein: 0.7 g

GARLIC AIOLI (THE BEST MAYO FROM SCRATCH)

I was first introduced to real French-style aioli when I worked at a little French restaurant in Pittsburgh. This is not your typical mayo. The punch of fresh garlic is intense, and once you try it, you'll want to slather it on just about everything. Using avocado oil also makes this aioli much healthier than any store-bought mayo. For this recipe, you'll need an immersion blender with the matching blending cup.

Using a microplane or zester, grate the garlic clove into a fine paste. Place the garlic in the blending cup that comes with the immersion blender. Then, add the rest of the ingredients, cracking the egg into the cup last so that you don't break the yolk. Gently insert the immersion blender into the cup, over the egg yolk. Blend the mixture for about 10 seconds, moving the wand of the blender up slowly as you go. The mixture will emulsify and turn into a silky-smooth aioli. Transfer to a sealed jar, and keep it in the fridge for up to 5 days.

12 oz (340 g) tomatillos

1 small white onion

1 jalapeño pepper, stem and
seeds removed

3 cloves garlic

1 avocado, peeled and pitted

Juice of ½ lime

½ tsp kosher salt

¼ cup (10 g) fresh cilantro stems
and leaves

MACROS *per* SERVING (2 TBSP [30 G])

Calories: 25 • Fat: 1.7 g

Carbs: 2.7 g • Net Carbs: 1.6 g

Protein: 0.5 g

AVOCADO SALSA VERDE

This is one of those "supersauces" that I use for just about everything. This fresh salsa is perfect with eggs for breakfast, great for snacking and delicious with a juicy steak for dinner. Once you try this, you'll keep going back for more. And the addition of the avocado brings some healthy fat and creaminess to this recipe, which makes it that much better (and better for you!).

Try pairing this with the Slow Cooker Carnitas with Ancho Chile (page 55).

Preheat your oven to broil. While it warms up, peel and cut the tomatillos and onion in half, removing any stems. Line a baking sheet with aluminum foil, for easy cleanup. Place the tomatillo and onion halves, cut side down, on the prepared baking sheet. Place the pan in the oven on the top rack and broil for about 5 minutes, or until the skins of the tomatillos are black and charred (you want them burnt). Remove from the oven and set aside to cool.

In a food processor or blender, combine the jalapeño, garlic, avocado, lime juice, salt and cilantro. Then, add the charred onion and tomatillos. Blend until smooth and then chill in the fridge before serving. You can also add the salsa to a jar and keep it in the fridge for up to a week.

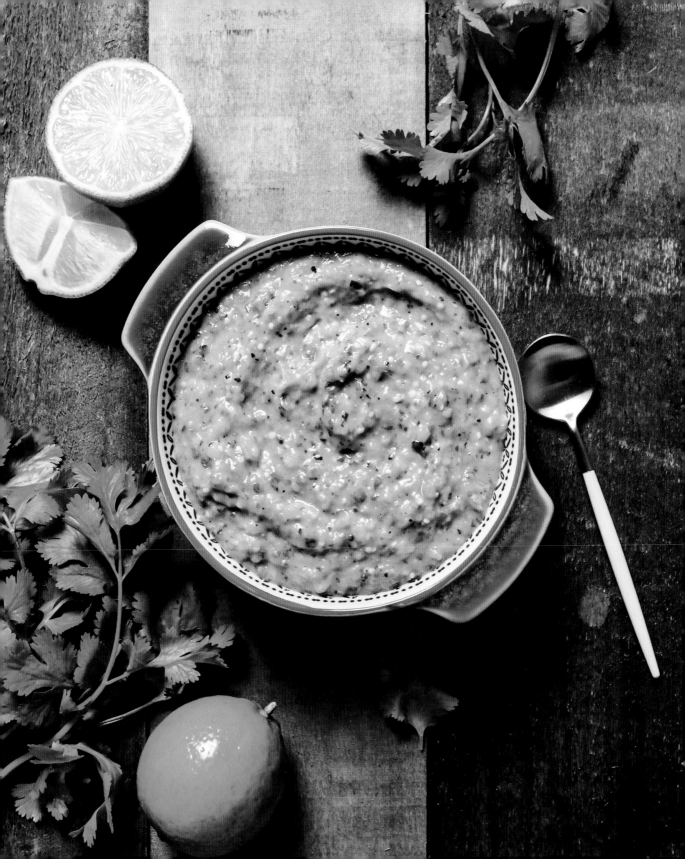

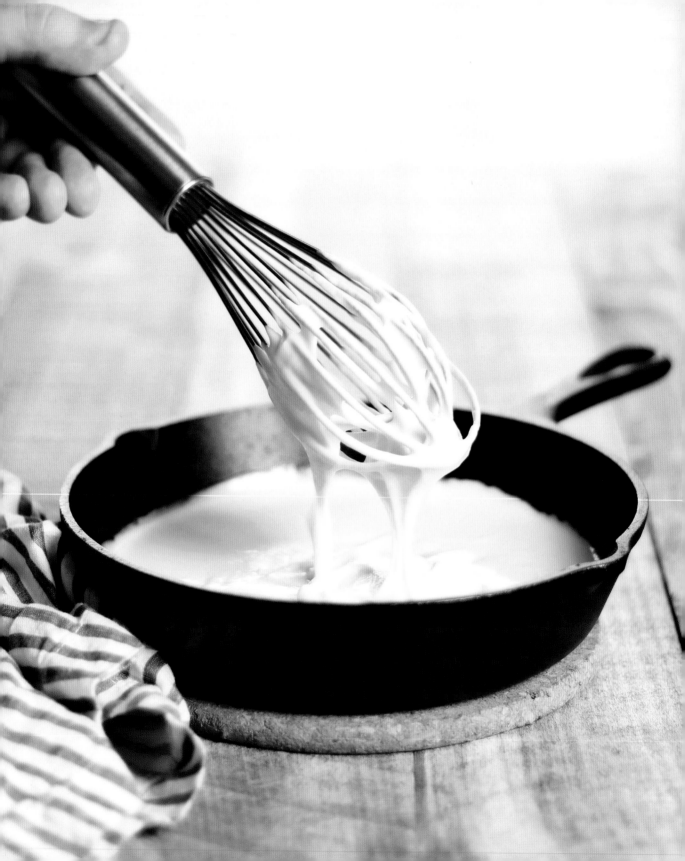

MAKES 1 CUP (240 ML) SAUCE

8 oz (225 g) Brie cheese

1 cup (240 ml) heavy whipping cream

2 cups (230 g) shredded mozzarella cheese (see Pro Tips)

MACROS *per* SERVING (2 TBSP [30 ML])

Calories: 265 • Fat: 24.7 g

Carbs: 1.3 g • Net Carbs: 1.3 g

Protein: 9.1 g

SECRET-INGREDIENT CHEESE SAUCE

I don't think there is anything more luxurious and decadent than this cheese sauce. The secret ingredient is the Brie, which makes this velvety smooth and extra-creamy. Smother your next steak with it, pour it over broccoli or cauliflower for a cheesy bake or add some chopped jalapeño to make the best queso ever. You can even use it with low-carb pasta for homemade mac and cheese. The possibilities are endless.

Try serving this on top of your favorite steak, tacos or even pasta.

First, carefully cut all of the rind off the wheel of Brie. Avoid removing any of the creamy center. Then, in a small saucepan, combine the Brie, cream and mozzarella. Place the pan over medium heat and slowly heat the mixture, whisking constantly. After a few minutes, the mixture will start to steam slightly, but do not let it boil. Once it's steaming hot, turn off the heat and continue to whisk aggressively until the sauce fully forms and becomes creamy, thick and smooth.

PRO TIPS: For the best results, shred your own cheese, as preshredded cheese is coated with starch to prevent sticking.

For a yellow queso sauce, use Cheddar instead of mozzarella. You can also experiment with adding other ingredients at the end. A few things I love to add are chopped jalapeños and ground beef, for a fun dip, or minced garlic and black pepper, which turns it into the most amazing Alfredo sauce.

Juice of 1 Meyer lemon (about 3 tbsp [45 ml] juice)

1 tbsp (11 g) Dijon mustard

1½ tsp (4 g) very finely chopped shallot

1 tsp herbes de Provence

1 tbsp (15 ml) cider vinegar (I prefer Bragg organic) or white wine vinegar

⅛ tsp kosher salt

¼ tsp freshly ground black pepper

1 tbsp (12 g) erythritol or allulose sweetener

½ cup (120 ml) extra virgin olive oil

MACROS *per* SERVING
(2 TBSP [30 ML])

Calories: 163 • Fat: 18 g

Carbs: 0.6 g • Net Carbs: 0.6 g

Protein: 0 g

MEYER LEMON VINAIGRETTE

There is nothing quite as nice as a homemade vinaigrette and the Meyer lemon brings a more delicate sweetness than a traditional lemon. This dressing is based on the classic method of making vinaigrette, but with a few of my own twists added to make it simple yet elegant. Not only is this lemony dressing delicious with salad, but it makes a fantastic marinade for chicken. Make a double batch of this, place it in a jar and store it in your fridge for up to ten days.

Try pairing this with the Secret-Recipe Whole Roasted Chicken (page 73), or drizzle it over grilled veggies.

In a bowl, whisk together all the ingredients, except the olive oil; you can do this by hand or with a hand mixer. Then, while constantly whisking aggressively, use your other hand to very slowly drizzle in the olive oil. Once you've poured in the olive oil, keep whisking for an extra minute to completely emulsify the dressing. You can use the dressing immediately, or store it in a jar. If the oil begins to separate, you can use the jar to shake it, or you can whisk the dressing back together.

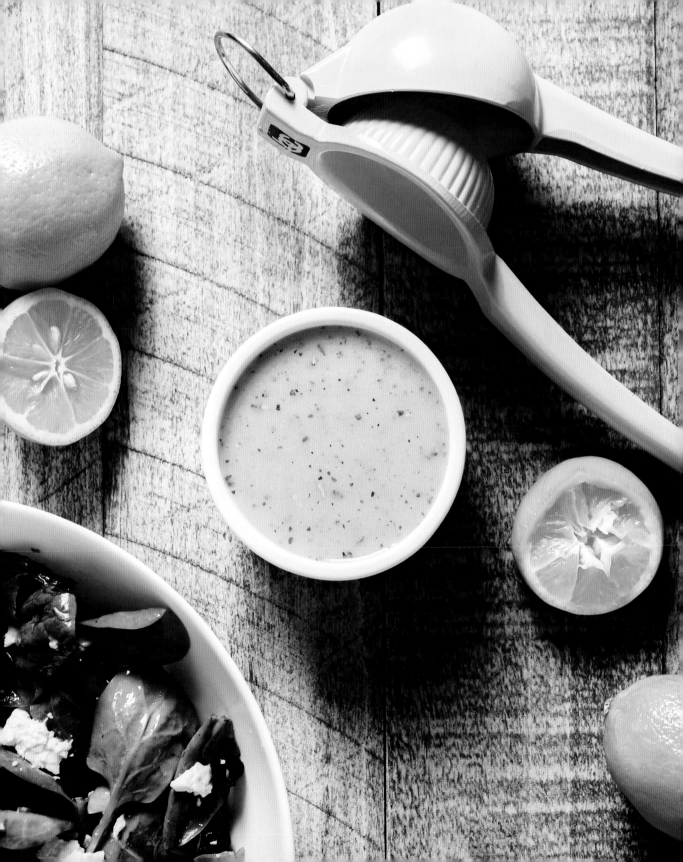

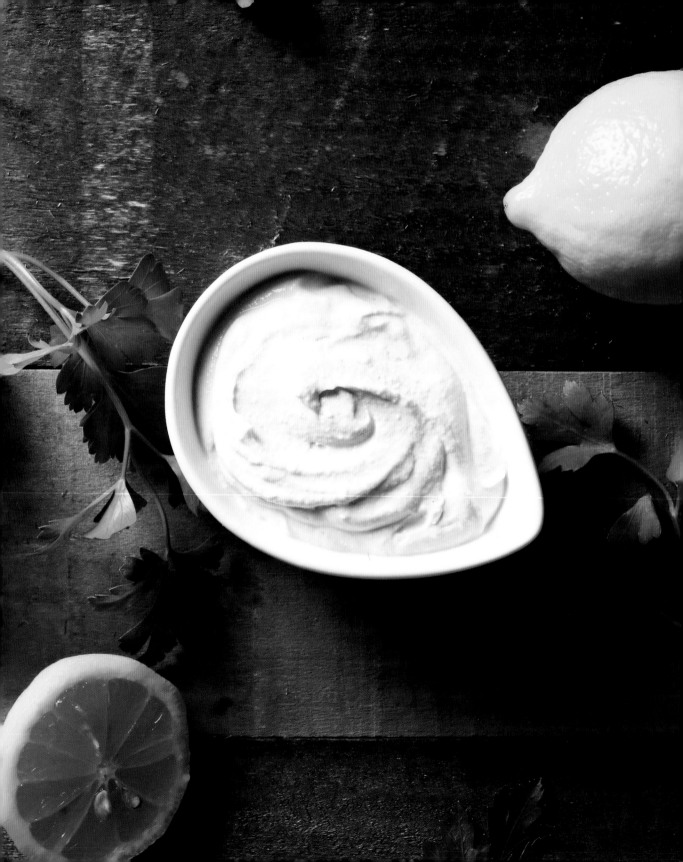

½ cup (120 g) 100% pure tahini

½ cup (120 g) full-fat plain Greek yogurt

Juice of ½ lemon

½ tsp kosher salt

4 to 5 tbsp (60 to 75 ml) warm water

MACROS *per* SERVING (2 TBSP [30 ML])

Calories: 104 • Fat: 8.8 g

Carbs: 2 g • Net Carbs: 1.5 g

Protein: 4.8 g

EASY TAHINI YOGURT SAUCE

This incredible sauce is only four ingredients (five, if you count water). Tahini is just ground-up sesame seeds, and it has the most incredible flavor. It works as a dipping sauce or salad dressing, and goes incredibly well with lamb, steak, chicken or roasted veggies. The nuttiness from the tahini goes perfectly with the tangy yogurt, and the sauce is packed with healthy fats and nutrients.

Try pairing this with the Za'atar-Crusted Chicken & Roasted Carrots (page 93).

In a bowl, combine the tahini, yogurt, lemon juice and salt. Then, add the warm water, 1 tablespoon (15 ml) at a time, until the sauce loosens and becomes smooth and creamy. The amount of water you will need depends on the tahini you have, as some brands of tahini are extremely thick and require extra water to loosen the sauce. You want it to be just thick enough to drizzle. Serve immediately, or save it in a jar in the fridge for up to a week.

½ cup (120 ml) sesame oil

⅓ cup (80 ml) soy sauce

⅓ cup (80 ml) olive or
avocado oil

6 cloves garlic

1½ oz (40 g) fresh ginger, peeled
and sliced (about a 2" [5-cm] piece)

2 tsp (8 g) Dijon mustard

¼ cup (48 g) allulose or
erythritol sweetener

⅛ tsp red pepper flakes
(optional)

Sesame seeds, for garnish
(optional)

MACROS *per* SERVING (2 TBSP [30 ML])

Calories: 220 • Fat: 23 g

Carbs: 1.8 g • Net Carbs: 1.6 g

Protein: 0.8 g

JAPANESE SESAME GINGER DRESSING

Not only is this an amazing salad dressing, but it's a must-try marinade for steak or salmon! The zesty ginger and nutty sesame create a perfect balance of flavor that complements whatever it touches. If you are bored of the same old marinades, this one is definitely for you. And this low-carb, high-fat version is perfect for your Keto lifestyle.

Try pairing this with the Hearty Grilled Steak & Kale Salad (page 33).

In a food processor, combine all the ingredients, except the sesame seeds. Blend on high speed for about 2 minutes, until the dressing is creamy. If you still see large pieces of garlic or ginger, keep blending until smooth. Top with sesame seeds, if using.

Use as a marinade with steak or fish or as a delicious salad dressing. You can keep it in the fridge for up to a week.

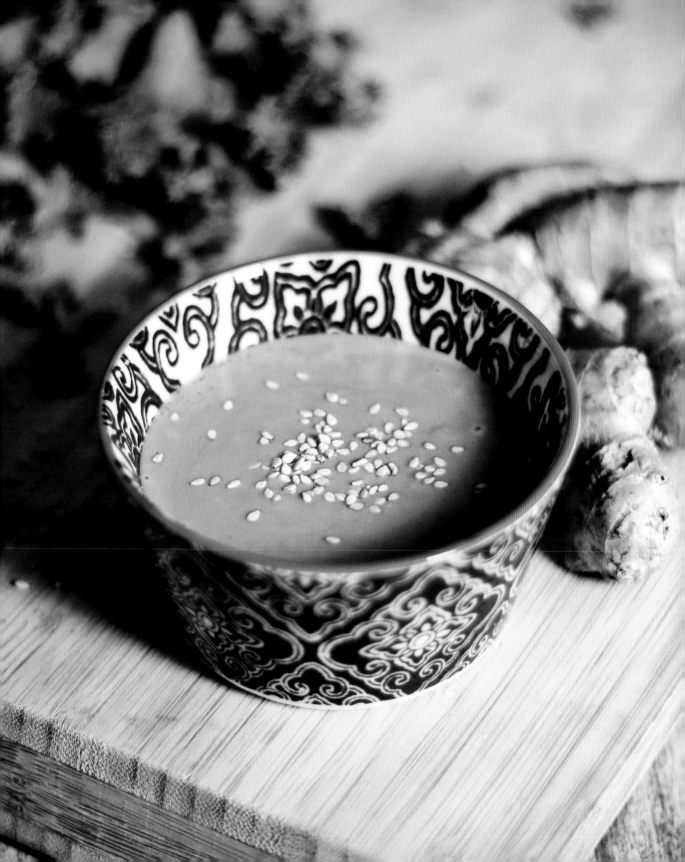

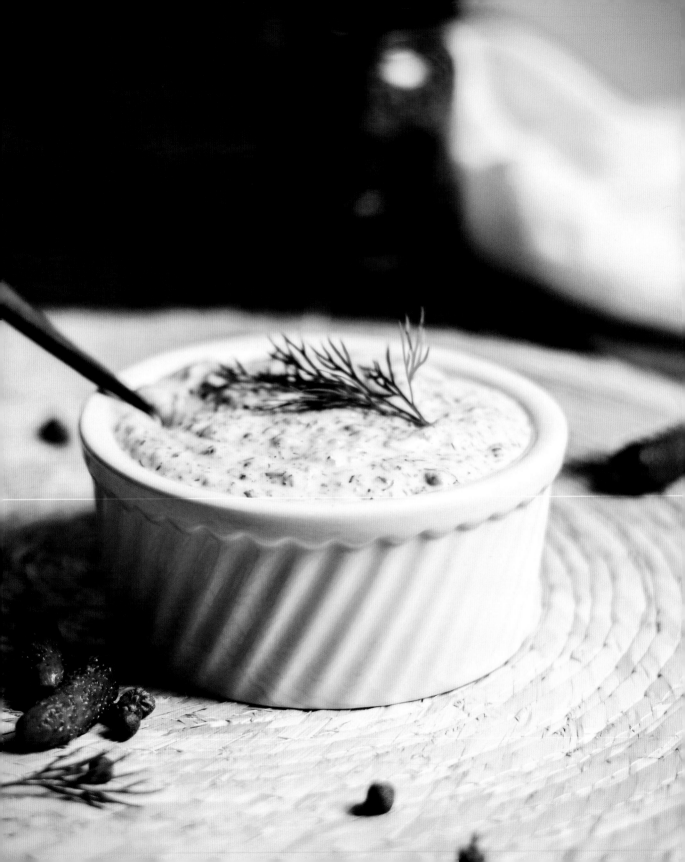

ZESTY DILL RÉMOULADE

This creamy sauce is basically the most delicious homemade tartar sauce. The cornichon pickles and capers give it a salty bite, while the horseradish provides subtle tang and heat. Try this with seafood, steak or chicken. Or spread it on your next sandwich for an extra kick.

Try pairing this with Mike's Signature Crab Cakes (page 70).

---

1 cup (225 g) mayonnaise

¼ oz (7 g) fresh dill, thick stems removed, plus more for serving (optional)

3 tbsp (26 g) capers

Scant 4 oz (50 g) cornichons or gherkins (about 10 pickles)

1 tbsp (11 g) whole-grain Dijon mustard (I recommend Maille "Old Style")

1 tsp prepared horseradish

In a food processor, combine all the ingredients. Blend on high speed just until no more large pieces are visible. Pour it into a jar to save it in the refrigerator for up to a week, or serve it in a bowl garnished with extra dill.

MACROS *per* SERVING (2 TBSP [30 ML])

Calories: 186 • Fat: 20.2 g

Carbs: 0.3 g • Net Carbs: 0.3 g

Protein: 0.3 g

½ cup (112 g or 1 stick)
unsalted butter

1 cup (192 g) allulose sweetener

1 tsp ground cinnamon

MACROS *per* SERVING
(2 TBSP [30 ML])

Calories: 103 • Fat: 11.5 g

Carbs: 0.3 g • Net Carbs: 0.2 g

Protein: 0.1 g

CINNAMON CARAMEL SAUCE

You will not believe this ooey-gooey caramel sauce is sugar-free and nearly zero carb. It is heavenly over ice cream, cake or even waffles! And it's totally guilt-free. For this three-ingredient recipe, you must use allulose as the sweetener. Other sweeteners will not caramelize properly.

Try pairing this with the Buttery Ghee Pound Cake (page 131).

In a small saucepan over medium heat, melt the butter. Once fully melted, add the allulose and cinnamon. Using a whisk, gently combine the ingredients. As the mixture heats up, the allulose will begin to dissolve. Once the mixture is melted, stop stirring, and do not walk away; timing is everything in this recipe. The sauce will slowly begin to bubble. After about 5 minutes, the bubbles will take over and start rapidly bubbling evenly across the pan (it will look foamy). Immediately remove the pot from the heat, then whisk constantly for at least 1 to 2 minutes. Let cool for 5 to 10 minutes. It will thicken as it cools. Use immediately while it's still slightly warm, or store it in a jar in the fridge for up to 10 days. Note: Once it has been in the fridge, you'll have to warm it up again to soften it.

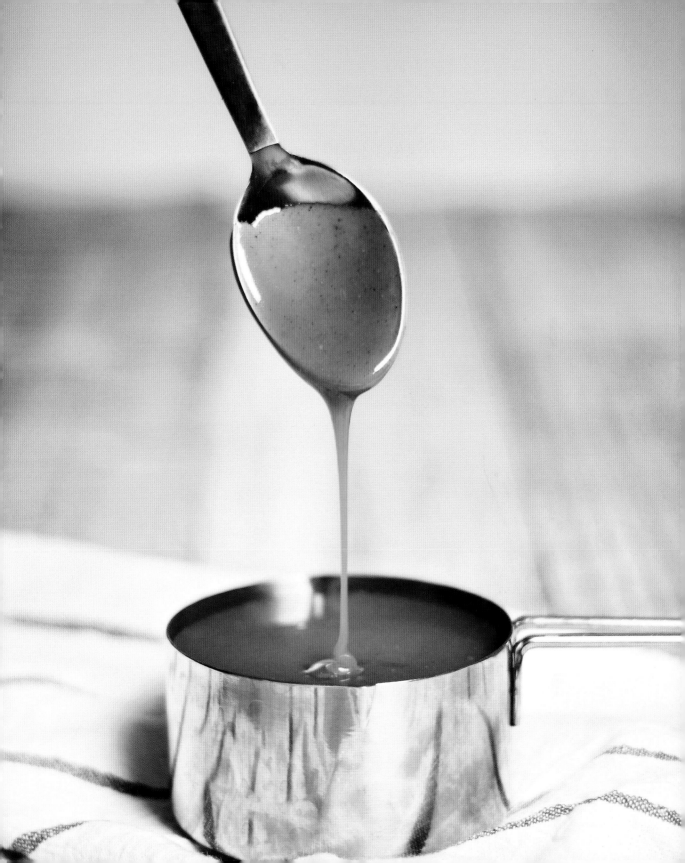

SALT GUIDE:

Iodized Table Salt:

High in sodium. Terrible in taste. Have you ever tried it plain? Yuck! It's best to avoid using this in your kitchen.

Kosher Salt:

Low salinity, tasty, and very inexpensive, kosher salt is the go-to salt for chefs in restaurant kitchens. It has the perfect-size flake to stick to raw meats and veggies and is the easiest salt to cook with. What it lacks in mineral content, it makes up for in consistency, usability and flavor. I recommend buying a box of *Morton's Kosher Salt* for your kitchen.

Sea Salt:

Packed with trace elements and minerals, sea salt has high salinity and good flavor, and it's a great all-around option for cooking. It's also the most nutritious, but it varies greatly across brands, which can make it unpredictable for cooking.

Finishing Salt:

These should only be used *after* a dish is done cooking. You may find high-end finishing salts, like smoked salt, black volcanic salts from Hawaii or Flor de Sel from the coast of France. These are to be used sparingly and are particularly tasty over a beautifully cooked steak.

Meat Temperature Guide:

BEEF	
Steak (flank, strip, ribeye, porterhouse, T-bone)	130°F (54°C)
Filet Mignon	125°F (52°C)
Prime Rib	120°F (49°C)
Meatloaf	160°F (71°C)
Burgers	135°F (57°C)

PORK	
Chops	140°F (60°C)
Tenderloin	130°F (54°C)

CHICKEN	
All Chicken	165°F (74°C)

FISH	
Salmon	120°F (49°C)
All Other Fish	140°F (60°C)

GAME MEATS	
Lamb	125°F (52°C)
Duck Breast	130°F (54°C)
Veal	135°F (57°C)
Rabbit	145°F (63°C)
Venison	135°F (57°C)

*Note: These temperatures are for medium-rare. Add or subtract 5°F if you want it more medium or more rare.

Cooking Fats & Oils:

	SMOKE POINT	SUGGESTED USE	FLAVOR
Butter	302°F (150°C)	Low-heat frying, sauces, baking	Creamy, nutty
Ghee	482°F (250°C)	Frying veggies, searing meat, curries	Cheesy, bold
Vegetable, Peanut and Seed Oils	400-453°F (204-234°C)	Baking, deep frying	Mild
Avocado Oil	520°F (271°C)	High-heat frying, searing meat, sautéing	Mild, slightly bitter
Olive Oil	320°F (160°C)	Roasting veggies and chicken, pesto, dressings, marinades	Fruity, spicy, flavorful
Animal Fat (bacon fat, lard, tallow)	370-400°F (188-204°C)	Roasting, sautéing, deep frying	Flavorful, complex
Coconut Oil	350°F (177°C)	Sautéing, curries, baking	Coconut
Sesame Oil	350°F (177°C)	Asian cuisine, dressings, marinades	Intense, nutty

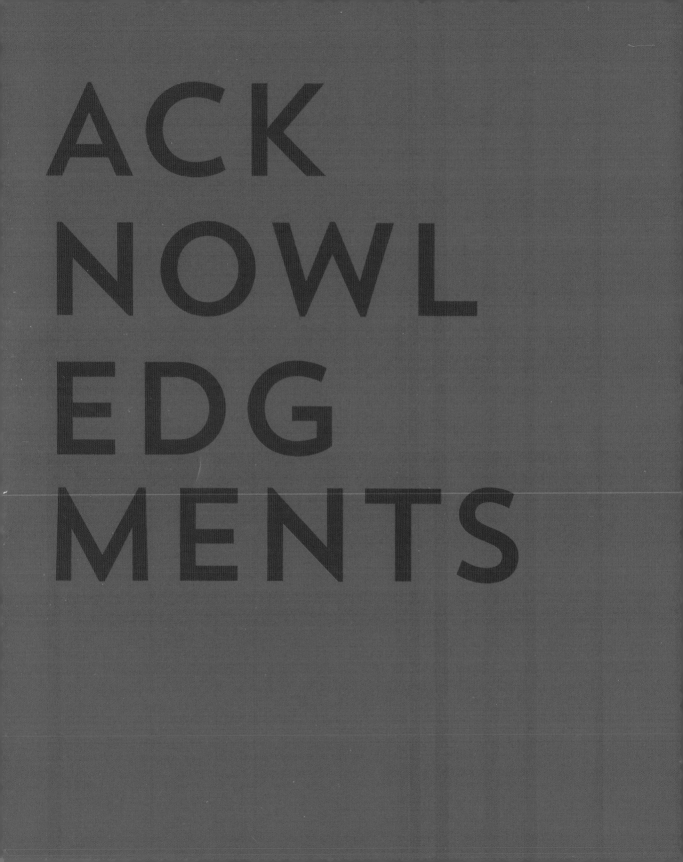

ACK
NOWL
EDG
MENTS

Indeed, it takes a village and this certainly did not happen alone.

Thank you to my family. Your love and encouragement has been my guiding light. Thank you to my amazing mother, who first sparked my love of cooking and has been an inspiration to me my entire life. Thank you to my brilliant father, who is the best person in the world to call for advice, and who's taught me everything I know about photography and so much more. To my big sisters, Jaimee and Laura, thank you for your friendship, support and wisdom. I love you all so much, and I owe everything to you.

Special thanks to Sanyu Kyeyune. Your insight and guidance has been truly immeasurable, and I couldn't have done this without you.

Thank you Caitlin, Meg, Will and the Page Street team for making this all possible. I am so grateful for everything you do and for giving me a chance to share my food.

Tess Kamban, Timmy Craig, Carolina Ramos and Milton Mejia, thank you for believing in me more than I believed in myself.

To my dear friends who have helped me through a crazy time, you have no idea how much it means to me, and I'll never forget it. Cheers to many more long phone calls and even longer hugs.

Thank you to the entire Keto community for becoming my extended family. You inspire me every day!

And thank you to Jacob, my heart and soul, who has put up with me for over a decade. You're a patient man. I love you.

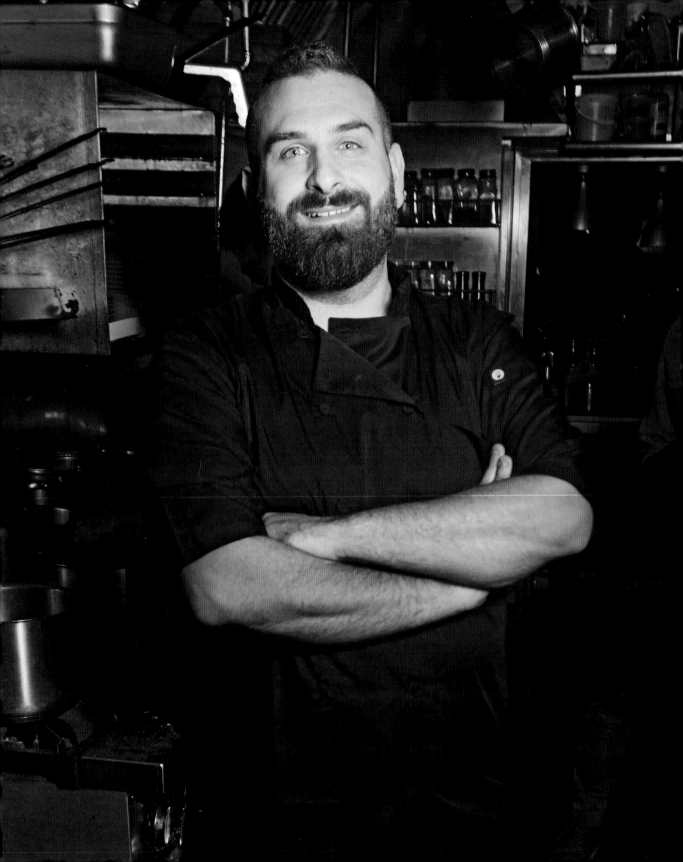

ABOUT THE AUTHOR

As a recipe developer, blogger and lover of all things food, Chef Michael Silverstein is passionate about the power of cooking to improve one's life. After beating out tens of thousands of competitors on Season 10 of *MasterChef* on FOX, Chef Michael has secured his spot as one of the best cooks in America. He is enthusiastic about teaching others how to cook healthy, delicious meals and firmly believes that anyone can make incredible food at home.

After losing more than 80 pounds (36 kg) in one year on the Ketogenic diet, Michael hopes to continue sharing his message that Keto food is beautiful. And while Keto is a powerful weight loss tool, he also believes that the benefits of a low-carb lifestyle are much more extensive than weight loss alone and works hard to create food that anyone would love, regardless of their nutritional goals.

Michael has a bachelor of science degree in business from Carnegie Mellon University. When he's not in the kitchen, he enjoys biking, playing piano, traveling and exploring the Austin food scene. He spends his free time at home with his fiancé, Jacob, and their rescue dog and cat.

For more of his recipes, find Michael on Instagram @chefmichael.keto, or on his website www.chef-michael.com.

INDEX

A

almonds and almond flour
  Buttery Ghee Pound Cake, 131
  Chocolate Peanut Butter Pie, 128
  Fluffy "Churro" Donuts, 127
  Hearty Grilled Steak & Kale Salad, 33
  Key Lime Cheesecake, 124
  Spiced Carrot Cake with Cardamom Cream Cheese Frosting, 119
Ancho Chile, Slow Cooker Carnitas with, 55
Argentinean Skirt Steak, Juicy, & Chimichurri, 51
asparagus
  Asparagus & Goat Cheese Frittata, 14
  Creamy Sun-Dried Tomato Chicken, 59
  Grilled Asparagus with Feta & Pistachio, 98
  Lemon Caper Shrimp & Avocado, 47
Asparagus, Grilled, with Feta & Pistachio, 98
Asparagus & Goat Cheese Frittata, 14
Avocado, Lemon Caper Shrimp &, 47
Avocado Salsa Verde, 55, 142

B

bacon
  Cheesy Brussels Sprout Gratin, 102
  The Chicken-Bacon-Mushroom Skillet, 52
  Crispy-Skin Salmon with Brown Butter & Pancetta, 74
  Mike's Signature Crab Cakes, 70
Bangkok Chicken Satay with Peanut Sauce, 29
"Banh Mi" Lettuce Wraps, Vietnamese, 34
beef
  Black Pepper Braised Short Ribs, 82
  Filet Mignon with Warm Spinach & Balsamic Reduction, 77
  Juicy Argentinean Skirt Steak & Chimichurri, 51
  Korean Beef Bulgogi Ssam, 89
  Seared Ribeye with Blue Cheese & Chive Compound Butter, 44
  Stacked Breakfast Tostadas, 17
  temperature guide, 157
Beef Bulgogi Ssam, Korean, 89
bell peppers
  Butternut Squash & Chorizo Hash, 22
  Shrimp Fajitas with Chipotle Crema, 26
  Spicy Sausage & Feta Shakshuka, 21
Berry Cheesecake Trifle, 116
blackberries
  Berry Cheesecake Trifle, 116
Black Pepper Braised Short Ribs, 82
blueberries
  Berry Cheesecake Trifle, 116
Blue Cheese & Chive Compound Butter, Seared Ribeye with, 44
Boursin-Stuffed Chicken, 37
Brie cheese
  Secret-Ingredient Cheese Sauce, 145
Broccolini, Lemony Charred, 106
brunch
  Asparagus & Goat Cheese Frittata, 14

Butternut Squash & Chorizo Hash, 22
Parmesan Prosciutto Tartlets, 18
Spicy Sausage & Feta Shakshuka, 21
Stacked Breakfast Tostadas, 17
Brussels Sprout Gratin, Cheesy, 102
Brussels sprouts
  Cheesy Brussels Sprout Gratin, 102
  Mediterranean Roasted Salmon & Brussels Sprouts, 43
Butter, Blue Cheese & Chive Compound, 44
Butternut Squash & Chorizo Hash, 22
Buttery Ghee Pound Cake, 131
Button Mushroom Flambé, 110

C

cabbage
  Hearty Grilled Steak & Kale Salad, 33
  Jicama & Orange Slaw, 113
  Seared Snapper with Wine-Braised Red Cabbage, 90
Caper Shrimp, Lemon, & Avocado, 47
Caramel Flan with Candy Tuile, 120
Carnitas, Slow Cooker, with Ancho Chile, 55
Carrot Cake, Spiced, with Cardamom Cream Cheese Frosting, 119
carrots
  Spiced Carrot Cake with Cardamom Cream Cheese Frosting, 119

Vietnamese "Banh Mi" Lettuce Wraps, 34

Za'atar-Crusted Chicken & Roasted Carrots, 93

cauliflower rice

The Ultimate Creamy "Risotto," 109

celery root

The Perfect Mashed "Faux-tatoes," 101

Charred Broccolini, Lemony, 106

cheese. See also cream cheese

Asparagus & Goat Cheese Frittata, 14

Boursin-Stuffed Chicken, 37

Butternut Squash & Chorizo Hash, 22

Cheesy Brussels Sprout Gratin, 102

The Chicken-Bacon-Mushroom Skillet, 52

Creamy Sun-Dried Tomato Chicken, 59

Grilled Asparagus with Feta & Pistachio, 98

Instant Pot Paneer Korma, 67

Parmesan Prosciutto Tartlets, 18

Roasted Lamb Rack with Creamy Feta Sauce, 78

Seared Ribeye with Blue Cheese & Chive Compound Butter, 44

Secret-Ingredient Cheese Sauce, 145

Spicy Sausage & Feta Shakshuka, 21

Stacked Breakfast Tostadas, 17

Tiramisu Mousse, 135

The Ultimate Creamy "Risotto," 109

Cheesecake, Key Lime, 124

Cheese Sauce, Secret-Ingredient, 145

Cheesy Brussels Sprout Gratin, 102

chicken

Bangkok Chicken Satay with Peanut Sauce, 29

Boursin-Stuffed Chicken, 37

The Chicken-Bacon-Mushroom Skillet, 52

Creamy Sun-Dried Tomato Chicken, 59

Grilled Chicken Shawarma with Dill Yogurt Sauce, 60

Moroccan Chicken Tagine, 86

Rosemary Dijon Chicken & Haricots Verts, 40

Secret-Recipe Whole Roasted Chicken, 73

temperature guide, 157

Za'atar-Crusted Chicken & Roasted Carrots, 93

Chicken, Boursin-Stuffed, 37

Chicken-Bacon-Mushroom Skillet, The, 52

Chicken Satay, Bangkok, with Peanut Sauce, 29

Chicken Tagine, Moroccan, 86

Chimichurri, Juicy Argentinean Skirt Steak &, 51

Chimichurri, Spicy Red, 138

chipotle peppers

Shrimp Fajitas with Chipotle Crema, 26

Spicy Red Chimichurri, 138

Chocolate Peanut Butter Pie, 128

Chorizo, Butternut Squash &, Hash, 22

cilantro

Avocado Salsa Verde, 142

Slow Cooker Carnitas with Ancho Chile, 55

Spicy Red Chimichurri, 138

Vietnamese "Banh Mi" Lettuce Wraps, 34

Cinnamon Caramel Sauce, 154

Cinnamon Whipped Cream Frosting, 131

coconut cream

Bangkok Chicken Satay with Peanut Sauce, 29

Instant Pot Paneer Korma, 67

Pork Chops with Creamy Mushroom Sauce, 63

Rosemary Dijon Chicken & Haricots Verts, 40

coconut flour

Buttery Ghee Pound Cake, 131

Chocolate Peanut Butter Pie, 128

Key Lime Cheesecake, 124

Salmon Croquettes with Turmeric-Ginger Aioli, 56

Tres Leches Cupcakes with Cinnamon Whipped Frosting, 131

Coconut Tres Leches Cupcakes, 131

Cod with Charred Lemon & Braised Leeks, 81

Compound Butter, Blue Cheese & Chive, 44

cooking fats and oils, 157

Crab Cakes, Mike's Signature, 70

cream cheese

Berry Cheesecake Trifle, 116

Buttery Ghee Pound Cake, 131

Key Lime Cheesecake, 124

Spiced Carrot Cake with Cardamom Cream Cheese Frosting, 119

Cream Cheese Frosting, 119

Creamy Feta Sauce, 78

Creamy Sun-Dried Tomato Chicken, 59

Crispy-Skin Salmon with Brown Butter & Pancetta, 74

D

daikon

Vietnamese "Banh Mi" Lettuce Wraps, 34

desserts

Berry Cheesecake Trifle, 116

Buttery Ghee Pound Cake, 131

Caramel Flan with Candy Tuile, 120

Chocolate Peanut Butter Pie, 128

Fluffy "Churro" Donuts, 127

Key Lime Cheesecake, 124

Spiced Carrot Cake with Cardamom Cream Cheese Frosting, 119

Strawberry Balsamic Ice Cream, 123

Tiramisu Mousse, 135

Tres Leches Cupcakes with Cinnamon Whipped Frosting, 131

Dill Rémoulade, Zesty, 70, 153

Dill Yogurt Sauce, 60

dinner. See also weeknight meals

Black Pepper Braised Short Ribs, 82

Cod with Charred Lemon & Braised Leeks, 81

Crispy-Skin Salmon with Brown Butter & Pancetta, 74

Filet Mignon with Warm Spinach & Balsamic Reduction, 77

Korean Beef Bulgogi Ssam, 89

Mike's Signature Crab Cakes, 70

Moroccan Chicken Tagine, 86

Roasted Lamb Rack with Creamy Feta Sauce, 78

Seared Scallops with Pea Puree & Prosciutto Crisps, 85

Seared Snapper with Wine-Braised Red Cabbage, 90

Secret-Recipe Whole Roasted Chicken, 73

Spice-Rubbed Pork Tenderloin with Orange Gastrique, 94

Za'atar-Crusted Chicken & Roasted Carrots, 93

Donuts, Fluffy "Churro," 127

E

Easy Peanut Sauce, 29

Easy Tahini Yogurt Sauce, 30, 149

eggs

Asparagus & Goat Cheese Frittata, 14

Butternut Squash & Chorizo Hash, 22

Parmesan Prosciutto Tartlets, 18

Spicy Sausage & Feta Shakshuka, 21

Stacked Breakfast Tostadas, 17

F

Fajitas, Shrimp, with Chipotle Crema, 26

fats and oils, cooking, 157

feta cheese

Asparagus & Goat Cheese Frittata, 14

Grilled Asparagus with Feta & Pistachio, 98

Roasted Lamb Rack with Creamy Feta Sauce, 78

Spicy Sausage & Feta Shakshuka, 21

Filet Mignon with Warm Spinach & Balsamic Reduction, 77

finishing salt, 156

fish and seafood

Cod with Charred Lemon & Braised Leeks, 81

Crispy-Skin Salmon with Brown Butter & Pancetta, 74

Lemon Caper Shrimp & Avocado, 47

Mediterranean Roasted Salmon & Brussels Sprouts, 43

Salmon Croquettes with Turmeric-Ginger Aioli, 56

Seared Scallops with Pea Puree & Prosciutto Crisps, 85

Seared Snapper with Wine-Braised Red Cabbage, 90

Shrimp Fajitas with Chipotle Crema, 26

temperature guide, 157

Flan, Caramel, with Candy Tuile, 120

Fluffy "Churro" Donuts, 127

French beans

Crispy-Skin Salmon with Brown Butter & Pancetta, 74

Rosemary Dijon Chicken & Haricots Verts, 40

Frittata, Asparagus & Goat Cheese, 14

G

Garlic Aioli, 90, 141

Goat Cheese, Asparagus &, Frittata, 14

green beans

Crispy-Skin Salmon with Brown Butter & Pancetta, 74

Rosemary Dijon Chicken & Haricots Verts, 40

Grilled Asparagus with Feta & Pistachio, 98

Grilled Chicken Shawarma with Dill Yogurt Sauce, 60

Grilled Steak & Kale Salad, Hearty, 33

ground beef

Stacked Breakfast Tostadas, 17

Gruyère

The Chicken-Bacon-Mushroom Skillet, 52

H

haricots verts

Crispy-Skin Salmon with Brown Butter & Pancetta, 74

Rosemary Dijon Chicken & Haricots Verts, 40

Hearty Grilled Steak & Kale Salad, 33

heavy whipping cream

Berry Cheesecake Trifle, 116

Buttery Ghee Pound Cake, 131

Caramel Flan with Candy Tuile, 120

Cheesy Brussels Sprout Gratin, 102

Chocolate Peanut Butter Pie, 128

Creamy Sun-Dried Tomato Chicken, 59

Fluffy "Churro" Donuts, 127

The Perfect Mashed "Faux-tatoes," 101

Pork Chops with Creamy Mushroom Sauce, 63

Rosemary Dijon Chicken & Haricots Verts, 40

Secret-Ingredient Cheese Sauce, 145

Strawberry Balsamic Ice Cream, 123

Tiramisu Mousse, 135

Tres Leches Cupcakes with Cinnamon Whipped Frosting, 131

Herb-Roasted Kabocha Squash, 105

I

Ice Cream, Strawberry Balsamic, 123

Instant Pot Paneer Korma, 67

iodized table salt, 156

J

Japanese Sesame Ginger Dressing, 33, 150

Jicama & Orange Slaw, 113

Juicy Argentinean Skirt Steak & Chimichurri, 51

K

Kabocha Squash, Herb-Roasted, 105

Kale Salad, Hearty Grilled Steak &, 33

Key Lime Cheesecake, 124

Korean BBQ Pork Belly, 64

Korean Beef Bulgogi Ssam, 89

kosher salt, 156

L

Lamb Meatballs, Spiced, 30

Lamb Rack, Roasted, with Creamy Feta Sauce, 78

Leeks, Cod with Charred Lemon & Braised, 81

Lemon, Cod with Charred, & Braised Leeks, 81

Lemon, Meyer, Vinaigrette, 146

Lemon Caper Shrimp & Avocado, 47

Lemony Charred Broccolini, 106

lettuce
Korean Beef Bulgogi Ssam, 89
Vietnamese "Banh Mi" Lettuce Wraps, 34

Lettuce Wraps, Vietnamese "Banh Mi," 34

limes
Avocado Salsa Verde, 142
Bangkok Chicken Satay with Peanut Sauce, 29
Key Lime Cheesecake, 124
Shrimp Fajitas with Chipotle Crema, 26

lunch
Bangkok Chicken Satay with Peanut Sauce, 29
Hearty Grilled Steak & Kale Salad, 33
Shrimp Fajitas with Chipotle Crema, 26
Spiced Lamb Meatballs, 30
Vietnamese "Banh Mi" Lettuce Wraps, 34

M

mascarpone cheese
Tiramisu Mousse, 135

Meatballs, Spiced Lamb, 30

meat temperature guide, 157

Mediterranean Roasted Salmon & Brussels Sprouts, 43

Meyer Lemon Vinaigrette, 37, 56, 146

Mike's Signature Crab Cakes, 70

Miso-Glazed Pork Ribs, 48

Moroccan Chicken Tagine, 86

Mousse, Tiramisu, 135

mozzarella cheese
Creamy Sun-Dried Tomato Chicken, 59
Secret-Ingredient Cheese Sauce, 145

mushrooms
Button Mushroom Flambé, 110
The Chicken-Bacon-Mushroom Skillet, 52
Pork Chops with Creamy Mushroom Sauce, 63
The Ultimate Creamy "Risotto," 109

O

onions
Avocado Salsa Verde, 142
Butternut Squash & Chorizo Hash, 22
Instant Pot Paneer Korma, 67
Korean BBQ Pork Belly, 64
Moroccan Chicken Tagine, 86
Shrimp Fajitas with Chipotle Crema, 26
Slow Cooker Carnitas with Ancho Chile, 55
Spicy Sausage & Feta Shakshuka, 21

Orange, Jicama &, Slaw, 113

Orange Gastrique, 94

P

Pancetta, Crispy-Skin Salmon with Brown Butter &, 74

Paneer Korma, Instant Pot, 67

Parmesan cheese
Asparagus & Goat Cheese Frittata, 14
Boursin-Stuffed Chicken, 37
Cheesy Brussels Sprout Gratin, 102
Creamy Sun-Dried Tomato Chicken, 59

Parmesan Prosciutto Tartlets, 18

The Ultimate Creamy "Risotto," 109

Parmesan Prosciutto Tartlets, 18

parsley
Juicy Argentinean Skirt Steak & Chimichurri, 51
Mediterranean Roasted Salmon & Brussels Sprouts, 43

peanut butter
Bangkok Chicken Satay with Peanut Sauce, 29
Chocolate Peanut Butter Pie, 128

Pea Puree & Prosciutto Crisps, 85

peas
Instant Pot Paneer Korma, 67
Seared Scallops with Pea Puree & Prosciutto Crisps, 85

Perfect Mashed "Faux-tatoes," The, 101

Pistachio, Grilled Asparagus with Feta &, 98

pork
Korean BBQ Pork Belly, 64
Miso-Glazed Pork Ribs, 48
Pork Chops with Creamy Mushroom Sauce, 63
Slow Cooker Carnitas with Ancho Chile, 55
Spice-Rubbed Pork Tenderloin with Orange Gastrique, 94
temperature guide, 157
Vietnamese "Banh Mi" Lettuce Wraps, 34

Pork Chops with Creamy Mushroom Sauce, 63

Pork Ribs, Miso-Glazed, 48

Pork Tenderloin, Spice-Rubbed, with Orange Gastrique, 94

Pound Cake, Buttery Ghee, 131

prosciutto
Parmesan Prosciutto Tartlets, 18

Seared Scallops with Pea Puree & Prosciutto Crisps, 85

Prosciutto Crisps, 85

Prosciutto Tartlets, Parmesan, 18

Q

queso fresco
Butternut Squash & Chorizo Hash, 22
Stacked Breakfast Tostadas, 17

R

raspberries
Berry Cheesecake Trifle, 116

red cabbage
Hearty Grilled Steak & Kale Salad, 33
Jicama & Orange Slaw, 113
Seared Snapper with Wine-Braised Red Cabbage, 90

Ribeye, Seared, with Blue Cheese & Chive Compound Butter, 44

ribeye steak
Korean Beef Bulgogi Ssam, 89
Seared Ribeye with Blue Cheese & Chive Compound Butter, 44

Roasted Chicken, Secret-Recipe Whole, 73

Roasted Lamb Rack with Creamy Feta Sauce, 78

Roasted Salmon, Mediterranean, & Brussels Sprouts, 43

Rosemary Dijon Chicken & Haricots Verts, 40

S

Salad, Hearty Grilled Steak & Kale, 33

Salmon, Crispy-Skin, with Brown Butter & Pancetta, 74

Salmon, Mediterranean Roasted, & Brussels Sprouts, 43

Salmon Croquettes with Turmeric-Ginger Aioli, 56

Salsa Verde, Avocado, 55, 142

salt guide, 156

sauces and marinades
Avocado Salsa Verde, 142
Cinnamon Caramel Sauce, 154
Creamy Feta Sauce, 78
Dill Yogurt Sauce, 60
Easy Peanut Sauce, 29
Easy Tahini Yogurt Sauce, 149
Garlic Aioli, 141
Japanese Sesame Ginger Dressing, 150
Meyer Lemon Vinaigrette, 146
Orange Gastrique, 94
Secret-Ingredient Cheese Sauce, 145
Spicy Red Chimichurri, 138
Turmeric-Ginger Aioli, 56
Zesty Dill Rémoulade, 153

Sausage, Spicy, Feta Shakshuka, 21

Scallops, Seared, with Pea Puree & Prosciutto Crisps, 85

seafood. See fish and seafood

Seared Ribeye with Blue Cheese & Chive Compound Butter, 44

Seared Scallops with Pea Puree & Prosciutto Crisps, 85

Seared Snapper with Wine-Braised Red Cabbage, 90

sea salt, 156

Secret-Ingredient Cheese Sauce, 145

Secret-Recipe Whole Roasted Chicken, 73

Sesame Ginger Dressing, Japanese, 33, 150

Shakshuka, Spicy Sausage & Feta, 21

Shawarma, Grilled Chicken, with Dill Yogurt Sauce, 60

Short Ribs, Black Pepper Braised, 82

Shrimp, Lemon Caper, & Avocado, 47

Shrimp Fajitas with Chipotle Crema, 26

sides. See veggies & sides
Slow Cooker Carnitas with Ancho Chile, 55
Snapper, Seared, with Wine-Braised Red Cabbage, 90
sour cream
    Key Lime Cheesecake, 124
    Shrimp Fajitas with Chipotle Crema, 26
    Spiced Carrot Cake with Cardamom Cream Cheese Frosting, 119
    Stacked Breakfast Tostadas, 17
    Tres Leches Cupcakes with Cinnamon Whipped Frosting, 131
Spiced Carrot Cake with Cardamom Cream Cheese Frosting, 119
Spiced Lamb Meatballs, 30
Spice-Rubbed Pork Tenderloin with Orange Gastrique, 94
Spicy Red Chimichurri, 138
Spicy Sausage & Feta Shakshuka, 21
spinach
    Boursin-Stuffed Chicken, 37
    Filet Mignon with Warm Spinach & Balsamic Reduction, 77
squash
    Butternut Squash & Chorizo Hash, 22
    Herb-Roasted Kabocha Squash, 105
    Moroccan Chicken Tagine, 86
Stacked Breakfast Tostadas, 17
Steak, Hearty Grilled, & Kale Salad, 33
strawberries
    Berry Cheesecake Trifle, 116
    Strawberry Balsamic Ice Cream, 123
Strawberry Balsamic Ice Cream, 123

summer squash
    Moroccan Chicken Tagine, 86
Sun-Dried Tomato Chicken, Creamy, 59
Swiss cheese
    The Chicken-Bacon-Mushroom Skillet, 52

T
Tahini Yogurt Sauce, Easy, 30, 149
Tartlets, Parmesan Prosciutto, 18
Tiramisu Mousse, 135
tomatillos
    Avocado Salsa Verde, 142
Tomato, Warm Spinach &, Salad, 77
Tostadas, Stacked Breakfast, 17
Tres Leches Cupcakes with Cinnamon Whipped Frosting, 131
Turmeric-Ginger Aioli, 56

U
Ultimate Creamy "Risotto," The, 109

V
veggies & sides
    Button Mushroom Flambé, 110
    Cheesy Brussels Sprout Gratin, 102
    Grilled Asparagus with Feta & Pistachio, 98
    Herb-Roasted Kabocha Squash, 105
    Jicama & Orange Slaw, 113
    Lemony Charred Broccolini, 106
    The Perfect Mashed "Faux-tatoes," 101
    The Ultimate Creamy "Risotto," 109
Vietnamese "Banh Mi" Lettuce Wraps, 34

W
Warm Spinach & Balsamic Reduction, Filet Mignon with, 77
weeknight meals
    The Chicken-Bacon-Mushroom Skillet, 52
    Creamy Sun-Dried Tomato Chicken, 59
    Grilled Chicken Shawarma with Dill Yogurt Sauce, 60
    Instant Pot Paneer Korma, 67
    Juicy Argentinean Skirt Steak & Chimichurri, 51
    Korean BBQ Pork Belly, 64
    Lemon Caper Shrimp & Avocado, 47
    Mediterranean Roasted Salmon & Brussels Sprouts, 43
    Miso-Glazed Pork Ribs, 48
    Pork Chops with Creamy Mushroom Sauce, 63
    Rosemary Dijon Chicken & Haricots Verts, 40
    Salmon Croquettes with Turmeric-Ginger Aioli, 56
    Seared Ribeye with Blue Cheese & Chive Compound Butter, 44
    Slow Cooker Carnitas with Ancho Chile, 55
Whole Roasted Chicken, Secret-Recipe, 73

Z
Za'atar-Crusted Chicken & Roasted Carrots, 93
Zesty Dill Rémoulade, 70, 153
zucchini
    Moroccan Chicken Tagine, 86